Neonatal Transfusion Practices

Deborah A. Sesok-Pizzini

Editor

Neonatal Transfusion Practices

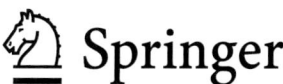 Springer

Editor
Deborah A. Sesok-Pizzini
Department of Pathology and Laboratory Medicine
The Children's Hospital of Philadelphia
Philadelphia
Pennsylvania
USA

ISBN 978-3-319-42762-1   ISBN 978-3-319-42764-5   (eBook)
DOI 10.1007/978-3-319-42764-5

Library of Congress Control Number: 2016958454

Printed on acid-free paper

This Springer imprint is published by Springer Nature
The registered company is Springer

This book is dedicated to the families of our patients, the families of our expert authors, and my own family as an editor and author of this book. Thank you all for teaching us patience and commitment to practice excellence while giving us the time and willingness to share our expertise with others.

Preface

Neonatal transfusion medicine is a distinct entity within transfusion medicine due to the unique features of the standards, practice, and biology surrounding these young patients. Unlike in adult blood banking, neonatal blood banking is much more of a boutique experience where products are customized to individual patients. This customization comes in the form of aliquot manufacturing, donor limitation, fresh whole blood use, and techniques including intrauterine transfusion and extracorporeal membrane oxygenation (ECMO). In addition, our neonatal patients have a unique set of disease management challenges including hemolytic disease of the newborn, newborn anemia and thrombocytopenia, and coagulopathy. Even risks for transfusion reactions may vary in neonates compared to adults with transfusion-associated circulatory overload (TACO) and hyperkalemia as a common concern for very small neonates requiring massive acute transfusions.

In this first edition of *Neonatal Transfusion Practices*, these expert authors cover the highlights of the practice including chapters dedicated to pretransfusion testing, manufacturing, standards, and storage; blood product administration; special congenital and acquired disorders in the neonate; hemolytic disease of the newborn; intrauterine transfusions; adverse reactions; and ECMO. A unique feature of our selected authors is that they are a diverse group of experts in the field and include pathologists, anesthesiologists, neonatologists, a pediatric hematologist and oncologist, and a high-risk obstetrician. These authors contribute their unique expertise and perspectives to the practice of neonatal transfusion medicine and allow the reader to experience an in-depth introduction to each of the chapter topics.

It is our goal with the first edition to create a "go-to textbook" for some of the more frequent questions we encounter from colleagues with more limited exposure to neonatal transfusion practices. From the safety of additive solutions to the preparation of products for an exchange transfusion to indications, dosage, and rates of transfusion of blood components, this book is intended as both an introduction and in many cases a more comprehensive guide to the practice of neonatal transfusion medicine. As colleagues, we are passionate about the care of our youngest patients and hope this book helps the reader appreciate some of the differences and challenges in transfusing neonates.

Philadelphia, PA, USA   Deborah A. Sesok-Pizzini

Contents

Contributors

Kelley E. Capocelli, MD Pathology and Laboratory Medicine, Children's Hospital Colorado, Aurora, CO, USA

Sara C. Handley, MD Department of Pediatrics, The Children's Hospital of Philadelphia, Philadelphia, PA, USA

Jaleah L. Hawkins, MD Hospital of the University of Pennsylvania, Perelman School of Medicine University of Pennsylvania, Philadelphia, PA, USA

Grace Hsu, MD Department of Anesthesiology and Critical Care Medicine, Perelman School of Medicine University of Pennsylvania, The Children's Hospital of Philadelphia, Philadelphia, PA, USA

Jamie E. Kallan, MD Department of Pathology, University of Colorado Hospital, Aurora, CO, USA

Nahla Khalek, MD Center for Fetal Diagnosis and Treatment, The Children's Hospital of Philadelphia, Perelman School of Medicine University of Pennsylvania, Philadelphia, PA, USA

Michele P. Lambert, MD, MTR The Children's Hospital of Philadelphia, Division of Hematology, Department of Pediatrics, Philadelphia, PA, USA

Perelman School of Medicine University of Pennsylvania, Department of Pediatrics, Philadelphia, PA, USA

Ursula Nawab Department of Pediatrics, Division of Neonatology, The Children's Hospital of Philadelphia, Perelman School of Medicine University of Pennsylvania, Philadelphia, PA, USA

Michael A. Posencheg, MD Neonatology and Newborn Services, Hospital of the University of Pennsylvania, Perelman School of Medicine University of Pennsylvania, Philadelphia, PA, USA

Deborah A. Sesok-Pizzini, MD, MBA Pathology and Laboratory Medicine, Perelman School of Medicine University of Pennsylvania, The Children's Hospital of Philadelphia, Philadelphia, PA, USA

Paul A. Stricker, MD Department of Anesthesiology and Critical Care Medicine, Perelman School of Medicine University of Pennsylvania, The Children's Hospital of Philadelphia, Philadelphia, PA, USA

Susan B. Williams, RN, BSW, RNC-NIC ECMO Center, The Children's Hospital of Philadelphia, Philadelphia, PA, USA

Chapter 1
Neonatal Transfusion Testing, Manufacturing, Standards, and Storage

Jaleah L. Hawkins and Deborah A. Sesok-Pizzini

Pretransfusion Testing

Pretransfusion testing is performed with the goal of identifying ABO/Rh grouping of the patient and donor blood as well as any clinically significant red cell antibodies against donor red cell antigens. This confirmation of donor-recipient compatibility is performed in order to reduce the likelihood of an immune-mediated hemolytic transfusion reaction.

The appropriate steps required prior to the start of pretransfusion testing will be discussed here as outlined in the AABB *Standards for Blood Banks and Transfusion Services* (30th Edition) [65]. Requests for transfusion products should be placed by a physician or other authorized healthcare provider with two independent patient identifiers. In addition, date and time of collection must also be recorded. All patient samples must then be received with sufficient identification, including two independent identifiers affixed to the sample container. Transfusion services must then confirm that all identifying information is legible, complete, and in agreement with the request. Patient samples and a segment of any red cell-containing component that has been distributed must then be stored in a refrigerator for no less than 7 days. In the event of an adverse reaction, this saved portion of donor sample can be used to for investigation [65].

J.L. Hawkins, MD
Hospital of the University of Pennsylvania, Perelman School of Medicine University
of Pennsylvania, 3400 Spruce Street, 6 Founders Pathology, Philadelphia, PA 19104, USA
e-mail: Jaleah.Hawkins@uphs.upenn.edu

D.A. Sesok-Pizzini, MD, MBA (✉)
Pathology and Laboratory Medicine, Perelman School of Medicine
University of Pennsylvania, The Children's Hospital of Philadelphia,
34th Street and Civic Center Boulevard, Room 5136 Main Hospital, Philadelphia,
PA 19104, USA
e-mail: pizzini@email.chop.edu

© Springer International Publishing Switzerland 2017
D.A. Sesok-Pizzini (ed.), *Neonatal Transfusion Practices*,
DOI 10.1007/978-3-319-42764-5_1

After identification and collection, special considerations for the neonatal population must be addressed in order to adequately assess appropriate donor products. Initial ABO grouping only requires testing with anti-A and anti-B reagents to determine the presence of A or B antigens on patient red blood cells. Reverse typing refers to the testing of patient serum for the presence of ABO antibodies. Reverse typing for anti-A and anti-B is not required in neonates since their immune systems are too immature to produce these naturally occurring antibodies. Rh typing is determined using standard anti-D reagent. Testing for unexpected red cell antibodies may be performed with either the mother's or neonate's serum.

Unlike the rigorous repeat type and screen testing in adults, limited repeat pretransfusion testing in infants less than 4 months old is acceptable by *AABB* standards [65]. Repeat ABO and Rh typing is not required for the remainder of the neonatal period up to 4 months of age; if the initial antibody screen is negative, the patient is being transfused group O or ABO identical RBC units, and units are either D negative or identical to the patient's D type [36]. Due to the immaturity of the neonatal immune system, it is unlikely that alloimmunization to red cell antigens will occur during the first 4 months of life [14, 47]. However if non-group O neonates (group A, B, or AB) are receiving non-group O cells incompatible with maternal ABO group, the neonate's plasma or serum must be tested for anti-A and anti-B antibodies. These test methods include antiglobulin phase testing using donor or reagent A1 or B red cells. If either anti-A or anti-B is detected, it is important to use red blood cells lacking the corresponding ABO antigen.

In addition, if the initial neonate red blood cell (RBC) antibody screen is positive, donor units lacking the corresponding red blood cell antigen should be issued. If there is difficulty identifying the antibody, it is advised that a sample of maternal blood be obtained for testing due to larger sample volume and more strongly reactive antibodies [62]. If the mother's sample cannot be obtained, cord blood samples may be used, if available. However, some laboratories discourage the use of cord blood due to concerns of test interference with Wharton's jelly. Subsequent to antibody identification, compatible units should be issued until the maternal antibody is no longer demonstrating in the neonate's serum.

Crossmatching

In urgent situations, uncrossmatched blood may be released if requested; otherwise, crossmatching or compatibility testing is required in the general population. In cases where all significant antibodies have been ruled out and there is no history of antibodies, abbreviated methods that only detect ABO compatibility such as immediate spin and electronic crossmatch or neonatal crossmatch can be applied [36, 65]. Immediate spin crossmatching involves combining patient serum of plasma with potential donor red blood cells at room temperature. After combining, the mixture must be centrifuged immediately. In the absence of agglutination, the donor and recipient are determined to be compatible. An electronic crossmatch is a computerized process where recipient-donor compatibility is verified based on patient serum antibody testing and ABO grouping. In infants less than 4 months old, compatibility crossmatching is not required for initial or subsequent transfusions if the initial antibody screen is negative [16]. If the initial antibody screen is positive, donor units lacking the corresponding antigen do not require crossmatch [65]. In some cases, the mother may have red cell antibodies prior to delivery. In this situation, identification of a compatible unit for the neonate may be challenging. Under these circumstances directed donation can be pursued if the mother is a suitable donor for the neonate. If maternal donation is not possible, or the antibody is against a high-prevalence antigen, other options including maternal sibling-directed donation or the American Rare Donor Program may be pursued. These neonates may be at risk for hemolytic disease of the newborn, and special considerations regarding red blood cell and component transfusions must be addressed [86]. These considerations are discussed in detail in Chap. 3.

Direct Antiglobulin Tests (DAT)

A direct antiglobulin test (DAT) may be performed routinely on neonates in tertiary pediatric facilities where neonatal care is very complex and a definitive diagnosis is obscure. Often, the neonate may show signs or symptoms of bleeding or hemolysis, and a DAT may help rule out maternal antibodies or hemolytic disease of the newborn (HDN) due to ABO incompatibility or other cause of hemolysis. This may also help guide early intervention of phototherapy or a need to perform a manual red cell exchange in the neonate. In many hospitals, it is not uncommon for a DAT to be part of the routine analysis of the initial neonatal type and screen. A DAT evaluates the presence of antibody on the surface of red blood cells. If this test is positive, an eluate may be performed. The process of elution involves stripping antibody from the surface of red blood cells using either freeze-thaw or heating techniques. Once antibodies have dissociated from the red blood cells, they can be identified using standard reagent cells [94]. Studies indicate that elution is more sensitive than DAT in detecting red blood cell antibodies; however, elution is not as widely available and can be labor intensive [92, 95]. There are some adult institutions with a limited neonatal population that do not routinely do eluates on neonates with a positive DAT. Instead, a diagnosis of ABO HDN or other hemolytic entity is inferred from testing maternal serum.

Aliquots

Current guidelines for pediatric transfusion recommend blood component dosing of 10–15 mL/kg for red blood cells and fresh frozen plasma. Lower dosages of 5–10 mL/kg and 1–2 units/10 kg are required for platelets and cryoprecipitate, respectively [100]. The small volume of blood components required by neonates poses specific challenges. Small-volume aliquots are utilized in many blood centers to provide the most appropriate product for the patient. A variety of methods are available to package blood components in smaller aliquots with minimal wastage of the remaining product.

The concept of aliquoting is based on the principles of sterile technique using pyrogen-free equipment [65]. Aliquots can be produced at either a blood center or hospital blood bank. Many blood centers institute quad packs produced from a single unit of whole blood. In this process, a primary bag of whole blood is attached to three smaller bags. During component separation, plasma is diverted into one bag, and the remaining red blood cells are diverted into the smaller bags. This entire process does not disrupt the integrity of the initial unit and is therefore considered a "closed system" that provides three aliquots from the same donor unit. These smaller packs can then be removed by heat sealer or metal clips and used as needed. This system is particularly helpful for transfusion services lacking sterile connection devices. In addition, this type of closed system allows maintenance of the expiration date of the initial donor unit. This method unfortunately can lead to wastage of blood components if the required dosages are smaller than the prepackaged aliquot [36, 73].

Other aliquoting methods including the production of small-volume transfer packs or satellite bags are often employed by hospital transfusion services [9]. The type of method used is oftentimes dependent upon the availability of a sterile connection device or sterile docking capabilities. When a smaller volume of component is requested, and the primary bags do not contain attached smaller volume bags, additional satellite bags can be attached to the primary unit either by "closed" or "open" system. The open method involves attaching a small-volume bag to one of the portals found at the top of the primary unit. The desired quantity of product can then be drawn into the attached small-volume bag. Although this system is simplistic and does not require the use of sterile connection devices, it produces risk for contamination of the original product as well as the newly produced small-volume unit. This results in a substantially shortened product shelf life for both the primary and satellite unit. The outdate is dependent on storage conditions. Products stored at 1–6 °C must be used within 24 h of preparation by the open method. Products stored at 20–24° must be used within 4 h [9, 65].

Closed system options are often employed by hospital transfusion services when a sterile connection device is available. Sterile docking allows the sterile attachment of two separate tubes without compromising the integrity of the primary unit. In this process, two equally sized pieces of tubing are heat welded together. Through this method attachments can be made between transfer bags, syringe sets, needles, and filters. Producing a sterile connection without sacrificing integrity produces several separation possibilities without reducing the shelf life of the final product. One such option is the use of syringe sets consisting of small-volume blood component bags or tubing with integrally attached syringes [20, 36]. This method provides an accurate closed blood delivery system based on volume per weight calculations. Some syringe systems offer an all-in-one set where the syringe is equipped with a 150u filter that completes the final filtration step required by the *AABB* Blood

Administration Guidelines, rendering a product that is ready for immediate use at the bedside [65]. The syringe system is considered accurate and can be used effectively to reduce both product manipulation and product loss. Currently, a variety of alternatives are available for the separation of blood and components by either an open or closed system. The aliquot method used is dependent upon the anticipated number of separations, method of separations, and the cost of materials. In the neonatal setting, syringe aliquots may be requested due to the need for strict volume control and the use of syringe infusion pumps [12].

In addition to providing the appropriate volumes of components with minimal wastage, aliquot systems can also provide limited donor exposure. Several studies have shown that assigning large volumes of blood components to a neonate for long-term transfusion support can substantially limit donor exposures during a protracted hospital course. After the initial product request and assignment, aliquots can be separated, dispensed, and administered over a long-term period [41, 44, 48].

Labeling

Once an aliquot is produced, it must be labeled appropriately to include the following information: unit of origin, expiration date, and identifier designating succession of each smaller unit. In addition, the date, time, identification of the person performing the separation, and lot numbers of materials used to prepare components should be recorded. The generation of a bar-coded label is also required by FDA regulations even if the aliquot is manufactured outside of the blood bank, e.g., the operating room. At minimum the barcode label must include the following: a unique facility identifier, a lot number relating to the donor, product code, and donor ABO/Rh type. This may be achieved by handheld bar coding devices which are available for purchase and can readily print a bar-coded label by scanning the original ISBT128 label [36, 89].

Blood Component Preparation and Separation

After collection, whole blood can be processed into three major components RBCs, platelets, and plasma by a variety of methods. All methods for the separation of whole blood components involve centrifugation as at least one step in processing. In contrast, apheresis-derived components undergo much less rigorous intermediate processing steps that will be discussed later in this chapter. Whole blood units are initially collected in 450 ml or 500 ml storage bags containing citrate-based anticoagulants [19]. The handling and immediate storage conditions of whole blood after collection varies based on the expected downstream preparation method and urgency. The most immediate step after collection is cooling. Blood left to cool at ambient temperatures cools quite slowly, requiring approximately 6 h to cool to a temperature of 25 °C. A study by Högman et al. [32] found that holding whole blood at ambient temperatures between 25 and 30 °C can result in profound loss of 2,3-DPG after only 4 h resulting in potentially impaired RBC oxygen-releasing function before collected blood is even processed [32, 66]. For this reason, many blood centers strive for more rapid cooling either by placement of collection bags in cool storage environments or with cooling plates that provide rate-controlled cooling at 20 °C. It should be noted that blood meant for platelet component separation should not be cooled to less than 20 °C as platelets are known to demonstrate optimal in vivo recovery and function when stored at temperatures between 20 and 24° [58]. In addition, the length of time that whole blood is stored is also dependent upon the intention of platelet separation and extraction method. Whole blood is held from 2 to 24 h after collection if the "buffy coat" preparation method is used, while other methods require platelet separation within 8 h of collection [19].

Platelets

Platelet separation can be achieved by two methods, either from "buffy coats" or from platelet-rich plasma. Both methods involve extracting the platelet component from an intermediary step during whole blood processing. A "buffy coat" is produced after unaltered whole blood undergoes a "hard spin" or a spin at high g-force. This separates the whole blood into plasma, red cells, and platelet-containing buffy coats. Buffy coats from multiple donors are then pooled together and centrifuged with low g-force ("soft spin"). This process produces a concentrated platelet product that can then undergo secondary processing such as leukocyte reduction, irradiation, or pathogen reduction. The buffy coat method is not currently employed in the United States [19, 28].

Platelet separation from platelet-rich plasma (PRP) differs from the buffy coat method in the sequence of hard and soft spins. The process is started with a soft spin that separates the whole blood into RBCs and PRP. The components are separated and then subject to a hard spin producing plasma and a platelet pellet containing at least 5.5×10^{10} platelets. The pellet can then be resuspended and sent for secondary processing, pooling, and/or storage. Plasma and red cells collected from the steps above are also subject to secondary processing and storage. After centrifugation and the removal of platelets and plasma, RBCs can also be resuspended in extended storage additive solution with a final hematocrit of 55–65 % [19, 28, 101].

Currently, most countries are in favor of the buffy coat preparation method [22]. Previous studies have found increased in vitro activation of platelets during the pellet stage of PRP preparation [28, 55, 81]. However, a difference in meaningful clinical outcomes associated with this in vitro activation has yet to be identified.

Once separated, platelets are suspended in plasma and must be stored between 20 and 24 °C under continuous gentle agitation for 5 days. Stationary storage of platelets has been shown to result in lactic acid production with subsequent decrease in product pH [18]. If agitation cannot be maintained continuously (i.e., during shipping between blood centers), interruption for a period less than 24 h is acceptable. Whole blood-derived platelets can be pooled from four to six ABO identical donors and are therefore referred to as random donor platelets. If pooling occurs in an open system, the product must be transfused within 4 h. If pooled using sterile methods, the pooled platelet units are maintained for 5 days under standard platelet storage conditions [19].

Bacterial Contamination

The storage conditions defined above put platelets at increased risk for bacterial contamination and proliferation, limiting shelf life to 5 days [37]. Bacterial contamination of platelets poses a substantial infectious concern with a reported risk of 1:1000–1:2000 units [7]. This is of special concern for the neonatal population given the immaturity of the immune system. Current *AABB* standards require routine bacterial detection methods validated by the FDA which usually include culture-based methods of apheresis-derived platelets or pooled donor units [25, 65]. Pathogen reduction technology has been routinely instituted in Europe, but has only recently been approved for use in the United States [65]. In the currently approved process, amotosalen (a synthetic psoralen derivative) is paired with long-wavelength ultraviolet (UVA) light to intercalate with bacterial nucleic acids, thereby inhibiting replication [99]. The procedure requires multiple steps where platelets are first suspended in 35 % plasma and 65 % platelet additive solution and passed through an amotosalen solution into an illuminator. After UVA illumination, the mixture then undergoes compound adsorption to remove amotosalen and residual photoproducts [43]. This pathogen inactivation method has shown to be effective against a wide range of pathogenic bacteria, viruses, and parasites. Unfortunately, the efficacy of the pathogen-inactivated platelets has yet to be elucidated. Multiple studies and meta-analyses have been performed comparing the efficacy of treated platelets with equivocal results. One such study by Abonnenc et al. [4] compared amotosalen-treated platelets to untreated platelet concentrates. Photochemically treated platelets exhibited "increased passive activation and moderate changes in adhesion and aggregation" [4]. It is still unclear whether these in vitro changes will be reflected in patient outcomes. The efficacy of treated platelets in the neonatal population is largely unknown. Concerns regarding the risk of hemorrhage have been raised. However, in the pivotal study evaluating the safety and efficacy of amotosalen-treated platelets, oropharyngeal bleeding and epistaxis were higher in the small group of pediatric patients compared to adults [91]. There may be a concern with treated platelets and increased risk of bleeding in the neonatal population; however, data is limited at this time.

Platelet Storage Media

Platelets are usually suspended in 40–70 mL of plasma. Multiple alternative options for suspension in saline or platelet additive solutions exist. However, in the United States, platelet additive solution (PAS) is only approved for apheresis-derived platelets. There are two platelet additive solutions licensed for use in the United States, PAS-C and PAS-F. Both types of solution contain chloride, acetate, and phosphate with differing concentrations of citrate, gluconate, and magnesium [1]. PAS replaces a considerable amount of plasma and has potential to provide increased benefit for plasma component-mediated transfusion reactions such as transfusion-related acute lung injury (TRALI) and potentially hemolytic transfusion reactions. It has already been associated with reduced rates of allergic and febrile nonhemolytic transfusion reactions [13, 87]. With regard to neonates, studies are ongoing to look at the safety profile for this product.

Plasma

Plasma produced during component separation is subject to a wide variety of storage, freezing, and secondary processing methods. Plasma is derived from whole blood via one of the separation methods discussed above or by apheresis. Most plasma is frozen shortly after collection and stored at subzero temperatures and thawed as needed. The time interval to freezing and secondary processing determines the storage conditions and shelf life of the final product as determined by the regional regulating body. The procedures discussed here are in accordance with the current guidelines and regulations set by the FDA and Council of Europe [19].

To be defined as fresh frozen plasma (FFP), plasma, either from whole blood or apheresis derived, must be frozen within 8 h of collection. Plasma can be rapidly frozen with various methods including blast freezers, dry ice only, or a mixture of dry ice and ethanol or antifreeze. Once frozen, FFP is stored at −18 °C or colder for up to 12 months. With FDA approval, FFP can be kept for longer than 12 months if stored at temperatures below −65 °C [65]. When ordered, plasma is then thawed at 30–37 °C in a water bath or by an FDA-approved thawing device. Once FFP has been thawed, it must be stored at a temperature of 1–6 °C and used within 5 days from the date of thawing or by the original expiration date, whichever is sooner [19].

Plasma frozen within 24 h of collection is referred to as plasma frozen within 24 h (PF24). Once frozen, this product is stored at −18° or lower for up to 12 months. The product is thawed by methods similar to those described for FFP and can be maintained for up to 5 days if stored at 1–6 °C after thawing.

Apheresis-derived plasma frozen within 24 h of collection that is first held at room temperature for up to 24 h is referred to as PF24RT24. This product is also stored at −18 °C and thawed with water bath or approved thawing device. Storage of the thawed products and expiration date are identical to that of FFP and PF24.

Thawed plasma is a derivative of either FFP, PF24, or PF24RT24. Once any of these components is thawed and held at 1–6° for more than 24 h, it must be relabeled as thawed plasma and continue to be stored at 1–6 °C for a maximum of 5 days after the date of thawing [1]. Currently, thawed plasma is not licensed by the FDA. Thawed plasma from FFP is known to contain reduced levels of Factor V and

Factor VIII. ADAMTS13 levels, however, are adequately maintained for the entire 5-day shelf life of thawed plasma stored at 1–6 °C [1, 19].

Plasma can also be classified based on the removal of cryoprecipitate. Reduced plasma cryoprecipitate is a by-product of cryoprecipitate antihemophilic factor separation from FFP. During the thawing process, insoluble protein precipitates can be collected by centrifugation. The supernatant is then transferred to a satellite container, and the precipitant is resuspended in approximately 15 mL of residual plasma and refrozen within an hour of removal. The precipitated product is known as cryoprecipitate antihemophilic factor, often referred to as "cryoprecipitate," and can be stored for up to 12 months from the original collection date at −18 °C. Current standards require that cryoprecipitate contains at least 80 international units of Factor VIII and 150 mg of fibrinogen per unit. In addition, cryoprecipitate also contains 20–30 % of the original Factor XIII and 40–70 % of the von Willebrand factor contained in the original unit of FFP [101]. The remaining plasma, often referred to as "cryo-poor plasma," although cryoprecipitate reduced, maintains normal levels of Factor I, Factor VII, Factor X, antiplasmin, antithrombin, protein C, and protein S. However, Factor VIII, von Willebrand factor activity, fibrinogen, and Factor XIII levels are reduced [19, 102]. Of note, methods of cryoprecipitate extraction often produce levels of coagulation factors that are much higher than the minimums listed here. Current manufacturing practices often produce fibrinogen levels greater than 200 mg [10, 19].

Despite the preparative method or the component indicated, sterile connections for the separation of components are the recommended approach for processing as this will allow maintenance of the primary unit's original outdate. Currently, fully automated systems for component separation and collection are available for performing the process in a closed system.

Another plasma product that is now available is solvent/detergent (SD)-treated plasma or Octaplas (Octapharma, Vienna, Austria). SD-treated plasma was approved by the FDA on January 17, 2013, but has been used in many countries in Europe for up to two decades. SD treatment is a pathogen reduction process where pooled plasma from up to 2500 donors is exposed to 1 % tri-n-butyl phosphate and 1 % Triton X-100. This treatment disrupts the lipid components of enveloped viruses such as HIV, HCV, and HBV. It should be noted that non-enveloped viruses such as parvovirus B19 can persist after treatment [25]. SD-treated plasma comes in standardized 200 mL units with a shelf life of 12 months. Units should be stored at −18 °C and should be used within 24 h after thawing. One of the challenges in the use of this process is the substantial reduction in functional protein S [19, 60]. For this reason, Octaplas is contraindicated in patients with severe protein S deficiency. This product is also contraindicated in patients with IgA deficiency or a history of hypersensitivity to plasma products. Excessive bleeding due to hyperfibrinolysis is also possible due to substantially decreased levels of alpha$_2$-antiplasmin [2, 101]. SD-treated plasma has been studied and approved for use in adult patients with liver disease, patients with thrombotic thrombocytopenic purpura (TTP), and patients undergoing cardiac surgery or liver transplantation. The safety and efficacy of Octaplas has yet to be established in pediatric populations. However, post-marketing studies are ongoing [90].

Red Blood Cells

After separation from whole blood or from apheresis-derived units, red blood cells are stored at 1–6 °C with a shelf life that ranges from 21 to 42 days depending on the combination of anticoagulant, preservative solutions, and secondary processing [65]. Anticoagulants and additive solutions are used for most red blood cell units for the preservation and extension of shelf life. Stored red blood cells are well known to undergo functional decline as well as metabolic waste accumulation attributed to a process known as "storage lesion." This widely studied phenomenon includes depletion of energy phosphates (ATP, DPG), dysregulation of calcium and potassium concentrations, the accumulation of reactive oxygen species, and membrane instability [21]. Additive solutions have therefore been developed to attenuate storage lesion effects by providing "volume for metabolic waste dilution; nutrients especially adenine and membrane protectant sugars" [11]. The additive solutions licensed in the Unites States have been shown to be safe in neonatal populations receiving simple transfusions [82, 83]. However, the safety of such solutions is controversial in neonatal patients with hepatic or renal insufficiency, those requiring massive transfusion, extracorporeal membranous oxygenation, and cardiopulmonary bypass [101]. Discussion of storage lesion effects and concern for fresher vs non-fresh red blood cells and outcomes is discussed more thoroughly in Chap. 6.

Anticoagulants

Current standards allow for a maximum of 10.5 mL/kg of whole blood to be withdrawn from donors. Care must be taken to avoid reducing donor blood volume too rapidly as this is known to cause severe reactions. With this in mind, 500 mL collection sets are available for larger donors, while 450 mL collection sets are preferred for smaller donors [19]. Anticoagulants are added in concentrations based on the size of the initial donor unit before processing with subsequent addition of extended storage additive solutions at a hematocrit of ~60 % [83, 85]. Approved anticoagulants include citrate dextrose solution formula A or B (ACD-A, ACD-B), anticoagulant citrate phosphate dextrose solution (CPD), anticoagulant citrate phosphate double dextrose solution (CP2D), and citrate phosphate dextrose adenine solution (CPDA-1). Currently ACD-A and ACD-B are not used in red blood cell units the United States. Approved anticoagulation systems base the concentration of anticoagulant solution on the size of the whole blood collection set. Table 1.1 defines approved anticoagulant formulations and concentrations for 450 mL and 500 mL collection sets. Of note, the addition of adenine to an anticoagulant such as in CPDA-1 extends the shelf life of red blood cells to 35 days. Therefore, red blood cells suspended in CPDA are maintained at a hematocrit of < 80 % and do not undergo further processing with extended storage media [19].

There are four additive solutions currently approved for use in the United States: additive solution 1 (AS-1), additive solution 3 (AS-3), additive solution 5 (AS-5),

Table 1.1 Approved anticoagulant formulations and concentrations for 450 mL and 500 mL collection [19]

Variable	CPD		CP2D		CPDA-1	
pH	5.0–6.0		5.3–5.9		5.0–6.0	
Ratio (solution/blood)	1.4:10		1.4:10		1.4:10	
Shelf life (days)	21		21		35	
Formulation based on whole blood volume	**450 mL**	**500 mL**	**450 mL**	**500 mL**	**450 mL**	**500 mL**
Sodium citrate, dehydrate (mg)	1660	1840	1660	1840	1660	1840
Citric acid, anhydrous (mg)	188	209	206	229	188	300
Dextrose, monohydrate (mg)	1610	1780	3220	3570	2010	2230
Monobasic sodium phosphate, monohydrate (mg)	140	155	140	155	140	155
Adenine (mg)	0	0	0	0	17.3	19.3

Adapted from AABB Technical Manual, 18th Edition

For 450 ml donations, donor blood is drawn into 63 mL of anticoagulant solution. For 500 mL donations, donor blood is drawn into 70 mL of anticoagulant solution

Shelf life days listed are FDA approved

and additive solution (AS-7). The formulations for each solution are detailed in Table 1.2. Concerns regarding the potential toxicity of additives such as adenine and mannitol have been raised in regard to renal and hepatic toxicity [33, 63, 71, 78, 84]. However, studies of additive solutions have consistently demonstrated that small-volume transfusions (10–15 ml/kg) transfused over the course of 2–4 h in the neonatal population do not result in deleterious effects on hepatic nor renal function. Prior study has shown that the concentration of both adenine and mannitol introduced into the bloodstream during transfusion of AS-1 and AS-3 RBCs falls well below the reported toxic doses of 15 mg/kg/dose (adenine) and 360 mg/kg/day (mannitol) [33, 78]. Similar low concentrations compared to reported toxic doses have been demonstrated regarding other toxic components in additive solutions such as sodium chloride, dextrose, citrate, and phosphate [45, 85]. Although previous studies have addressed the safety of additive solutions for small-volume transfusion in neonatal and premature infant populations, there is limited evidence regarding the safety of additive solutions for large-volume transfusions (>25 ml/kg) and in those populations with preexisting kidney or liver disease [33, 84]. Current guidelines for massive transfusions in neonates are based on case reports and case series and extrapolated from adult studies [15]. However, emerging evidence regarding the use of ECMO in neonates dictates that increased volumes of red blood cells are associated with worsening outcome in the neonatal population. Complications have been attributed to exposure to multiple donors and immunomodulatory effects

Table 1.2 The formulations for additive solutions approved in the United States [19]

Variable (mM)	AS-1	AS-3	AS-5	AS-7
NaCl	154	70	150	0
NaHCO$_3$	0	0	0	26
Na$_2$HPO$_4$	0	0	0	12
NaH$_2$PO$_4$	0	23	0	0
Citric acid	0	2	0	0
Na$_3$-citrate	0	23	0	0
Adenine	2	2	2.2	2
Dextrose	111	55	45	80
Mannitol	41	0	45.5	55
pH	4.6–7.2	5.8	5.5	8.5
Anticoagulant	CPD	CP2D	CPD	CPD

Adapted from AABB Technical Manual, 18th Edition
All solutions are FDA licensed

resulting in acute lung injury [57]. Unfortunately, the role that additive solutions play, if any, in these negative outcomes, has yet to be defined.

The lack of guidelines regarding at-risk populations and large-volume transfusions has led to a number of institution-dependent practices [72]. Some centers centrifuge aliquots of preserved RBCs followed by removal of the supernatant in order to achieve two major goals: (1) concentrating the RBC product to a hematocrit of ~80 % and (2) reducing extracellular fluid, thereby reducing the amount of additive solution. This method offers reduced concentrations of potentially toxic additives [85]. If larger-volume needs are anticipated, it is customary to resuspend the RBCs in plasma, albumin, or saline if appropriate. Some institutions may provide non-preservative units, where red blood cell products only contain anticoagulants (CPD, CP2D, and CPDA-1). However, this may require a special order that will increase turnaround time since the vast majority of units are preserved and CPD- or CPDA-only units may not be readily available. The use of non-preserved units is variable as a result of a lack of clinical trials to support or refute this practice. Anecdotal evidence suggests that the use of additive solutions for larger-volume transfusions is safe without reported adverse effects.

Apheresis-Derived Components

Although the technical process differs, apheresis-derived components are subject to many of the same guidelines as whole blood-derived products. All major blood components can be collected by apheresis methods, which are primarily based on a centrifugal technique. Apheresis-derived components are prepared from a single donor through an automated process. In this procedure, whole blood is removed from the donor and centrifuged by the automated device. The component of interest is then removed, while the remaining components are returned to the body in a continuous process. With the exception of platelets, the resulting apheresis-derived products can then be subject to the same standards, storage, testing, and secondary processing as whole blood-derived components [80].

Platelets produced by the apheresis method must contain at least 3×10^{11} platelets [65]. Unlike random donor platelets, the apheresis product is not pooled and is therefore often referred to as single-donor platelets. In addition, apheresis-derived platelets are approved for storage in platelet additive solutions which is designed to provide electrolytes and small molecules that support active platelet metabolism during storage [30].

Granulocytes

Granulocytes are typically used in patients with neutropenic sepsis who have failed treatment with antimicrobials. Granulocytes are derived by apheresis and must contain at least 1×10^{10} granulocytes suspended in 200–300 mL of plasma. In the neonatal setting, granulocytes can be prepared from the buffy coat of a fresh unit of whole blood if only a small volume is required. However, apheresis-derived products are preferred in both the adult and pediatric settings. Regardless of the preparation method, the product is stored at room temperature without agitation and should be used as quickly as possible, no later than 24 h after collection [9, 101].

Granulocytes are prepared by request requiring more stringent donor selection. Selected donors should be CMV seronegative (if the recipient is CMV seronegative), ABO compatible with the neonate, and negative for any unacceptable antigens defined by the antibody screen and patient history. The donor may require stimulation with steroid, granulocyte colony-stimulating factor (G-CSF), or both prior to collection. Due to the large number of lymphocytes present, secondary processing includes universal irradiation. Granulocytes should never be leukoreduced or administered through microaggregate filters [9, 101]. Currently there is insufficient evidence to prove the efficacy of this product and treatment with granulocytes remains controversial [56].

Whole Blood

The use of whole blood (WB) in pediatric transfusion is often reserved for cardiothoracic surgery or large-volume transfusion. Although not commonly available for allogeneic transfusion, whole blood can provide benefits for patients in need of red cells, volume expansion, and coagulation factors. Its use is commonly directed toward autologous donation in the adult population. Nevertheless, whole blood that is not intended for component separation is subject to the same practices and standards as discussed above. Whole blood is collected in 450 mL or 500 mL sterile, pyrogen-free containers with anticoagulant-preservative solutions to produce an anticoagulant-to-WB ratio as specified by the manufacturer. A 500 mL unit of whole blood has an approximate hematocrit of 40% and contains plasma, platelets, and white blood cells [5]. Secondary processing with leukocyte reduction filters can be directly applied to whole blood after collection. If whole blood is not intended for platelet separation, it should be cooled as soon as possible toward a temperature of 1–10 °C. Many practices accomplish this by using wet ice or other easily accessible cooling method immediately after collection. Subsequent shipping, cooling, and storage of WB should be performed by regional and nationally validated methods. WB should be stored at 1–6 °C within 8 h of collection. Once cooled WB can be stored from 21 up to 35 days depending on the type of anticoagulant-preservative used [19, 65]. Whole blood storage, unfortunately, does not allow for optimal storage conditions of its individual components. Alternatives to stored whole blood include both component therapy and reconstituted whole blood.

Reconstituted whole blood is the process of combining RBCs with ABO compatible FFP. The most common practice institutes in blood banks combines group O RBCs with group AB FFP. The Rh of both components should be compatible with that of the neonate. The goal hematocrit is $50 \pm 5\%$. Reconstituted whole blood can be stored for up to 24 h at 1–6 °C [20].

In adults component therapy is considered the standard of care; however, there has been a resurgence on interest in using whole blood in pediatric populations in the setting of massive transfusion. The original study of fresh WB performed at The Children's Hospital of Philadelphia showed that there was improved hemostasis and donor exposure limitation. The platelets at that time were suggested to be of benefit in these patients [49]. Other studies using reconstituted units also supported improved hemostasis and clinical outcomes in neonates undergoing heart surgery while significantly reducing the number of donor exposures compared to neonates treated with standard component therapy [27]. A recent retrospective analysis confirmed the reduced number of donor exposures [34]. Limited donor exposure may be of particular interest to parents concerned about transfusion-transmitted disease over the course of a long expected lifetime of a neonate. However whole blood transfusion is considered controversial. Despite prior study of WB in the pediatric setting, its use is not in widespread. The indications and use of whole blood are discussed further in Chap. 2. Of note, if whole blood is not leukoreduced with a platelet-sparing filter, it is important to obtain CMV-seronegative fresh WB in preterm neonates who are at risk for CMV infection.

Pathogen Testing

Despite the advent of multiple pathogen reduction methods, screening for infectious agents is a critical step in the blood collection process. A sample from each donation is screened for a number of pathogens. In the 1940–1950s, syphilis screening was the only test required by the FDA. The evolution of the screening process has been catapulted by the emergence of novel viruses to include a volunteer-only donor supply coupled with stringent viral, bacterial, and parasite detection methods. All testing is performed on samples collected at the time of donation. Platelets undergo an additional step in testing where they are cultured to detect bacterial contamination. This is generally performed at the component manufacturing facility. All US blood banks currently screen for the following pathogens: HBV, HCV, HIV-1/2, HTLV-I/II, syphilis, West Nile virus (WNV), and *Trypanosoma cruzi*. Most infectious disease screening is achieved by either antibody or nucleic acid detection. Antibody and serologic screening tests identify antibodies targeted against pathogens of interest with enzyme immunosorbent assays of chemiluminescent immunoassays. Nucleic acid testing (NAT) is now mandated in order to detect infection during the "window period," an early phase of viral infection where antibodies have not yet formed. Although these tests have shortened the window period, there is still an initial phase of undetectable viral infection. NAT assays were initially developed in 1999 to detect HIV and HCV infection, but now extend to include HBV and WNV detection. Repeated positive screens or a singly reactive NAT result leads to mandatory disposal of the donation [25].

Bacterial contamination of blood products can result in septic transfusion reactions. The source of bacteria is usually attributed to donor skin contamination. The pathogen burden is oftentimes too low to detect immediately after collection. However, replication can take place during storage, particularly in platelet components. Appropriate skin disinfection prior to blood draw is a vital step in the donation process. Separately the use of diversion pouches for the collection of platelet via apheresis or whole blood has been an *AABB* standard since 2008. In this process collection bags are equipped with a small diversion pouch that catches the first 10–40 mL of donor blood. The aim of this is to separate the donor skin plug from the final collection bag. As previously described bacterial testing of platelet products is required before product use [25].

Untested pathogens of concern include parasitic agents such as *Babesia, Plasmodium*, vector-transmitted viruses such as chikungunya and dengue as well as prion-mediated neurological infections. To date, there are no FDA-approved screening tests for blood donations. At-risk donors are detected only using the donor questionnaire.

Detection of cytomegalovirus (CMV) has posed a unique challenge within transfusion medicine. CMV is of particular interest in immunocompromised patients and neonates. CMV is a lipid-enveloped DNA virus that causes mild disease in immunocompetent individuals and persists as a lifelong latent disease. In the general population, 40–60 % of donors are seropositive for CMV antibodies [31]. Although routine testing is not required for every donation, CMV-negative donors are highly valued in certain clinical situations. While NAT testing is exquisitely sensitive for HIV, HCV, and HBV, its effectiveness is substantially reduced in CMV screening. This is the result of the virus' propensity for intracellular localization within white blood cells, namely, monocytes, as opposed to plasma [3]. Since latent virus survives in white blood cells, leukoreduction has become essential in high-risk populations such as low birth weight premature infants [6]. The practice of leukoreduction yields products that are termed "CMV safe" or "CMV reduced." However, studies suggest that secondary processing with white blood cell filters does not completely eliminate the potential for viral transmission [103]. The use of "CMV safe" products for neonates is variable across institutions and is quite controversial.

Some institutions prefer to serologically test for CMV virus in addition to giving neonates LR blood. This "belt and suspenders" approach to prevention of CMV infection is performed without a definitive clinical trial supporting this practice. A recent study at Emory evaluated CMV infection in neonates and determined the maternal breast milk was a significant source of CMV [35]. Other institutions will routinely give neonates LR blood as "CMV safe" blood citing the difficulty in obtaining CMV-negative donors, the low sensitivity and specificity of the CMV serological testing, and the lack of institutional evidence of adverse effects or increased CMV infection from this practice. In a recent AABB Committee Report regarding transfusion-transmitted CMV infections, no definitive evidence-based guidelines could be determined due to the paucity of data for the prevention of transfusion-transmitted CMV in current-day practice [3].

Of one exception may be intrauterine transfusions. A survey of AABB physician members revealed that many institutions prefer CMV-negative blood to "CMV safe" products in fetal and neonatal transfusions. Many academic and community hospitals will routinely provide CMV-seronegative donor products, resorting to LR products if the former is not available. Despite the lack of compelling data to support this practice, fetal and neonatal patients are the most likely patient population to receive CMV-seronegative products in the United States [79].

Component Modification

Leukoreduced Products

Donor units of RBCs and platelets typically contain as many as 10^8–10^{10} incidentally collected donor white blood cells (WBCs) [69]. The presence of WBCs in transfused products has been associated with a number of adverse events. Concerns regarding the suppression of the premature neonatal immune system have been raised [23]. Prior study in adults suggests immunosuppression associated with passenger WBCs following blood transfusion and subsequent increases in postoperative wound infection [97]. This may pose an increased risk for neonates who already have an immature immune system. Unfortunately, the study of the immunomodulatory effects of transfusion in the neonatal population is limited and not well understood [96].

The removal of WBCs has been definitively shown to prevent three major transfusion-related complications: (1) transmission of cytomegalovirus (CMV), (2) alloimmunization to HLA antigens, and (3) febrile transfusion reactions [54]. There is also some indication that leukoreduction (LR) may prevent other leukocytotrophic pathogens such as EBV and HHV-8, HTLV-I and HTLV-II, and *Ehrlichia chaffeensis* [69, 70]. Due to the paucity of studies in the neonatal population, universal leukoreduction of blood components in this population is difficult to justify. A Canadian study found no mortality benefit to universal leukoreduction of RBCs in low birth weight premature infants (<1250 g) admitted to the neonatal intensive care unit (NICU). However, LR-RBCs were associated with improvement in secondary outcomes such as retinopathy of prematurity, bronchopulmonary dysplasia, and necrotizing enterocolitis [23].

Currently there is no consensus regarding the risk of transfusion-related immunomodulation or its effects on nosocomial infection in pediatric populations. Despite the known benefits of LR in the adult population, it is not universally performed on all products destined for NICU patients. Canada and many European countries have instituted exclusive use of LR products. Those opposed to universal LR argue that many of the benefits are speculative and that further clinical trial is needed. However, there are limitations regarding the study of neonates that may prevent clinical trials from moving forward. Despite these arguments, the transfusion medicine community is moving toward universal LR.

LR is a benign process that can be started at any point after collection and can be performed at ambient or refrigerated temperatures [19]. Typically blood is filtered shortly after collection and before long-term storage. Filtering during earlier stages is thought to be beneficial since it removes leukocytes earlier in the process before substantial cytokine leak has occurred. In-line WBC filters are available as part of collection sets for both whole blood and apheresis-derived procedures. Filters can also be attached after collection using sterile connective devices. Bedside filter LR is also possible, though not the preferred method due to lack of standardization and quality control. Current standards require that leukoreduction methods decrease leukocyte counts to less than 5×10^6 for red blood cells and apheresis-derived platelets and to less than 8.3×10^5 for whole blood-derived platelets [65]. In red cells, the reduced product should contain at least 85 % of the original red cell content. For WB-derived platelets, at least 75 % of the units must contain >5.5×10^{10} platelets per unit [19].

Irradiated Products

Irradiation of blood products is performed to prevent transfusion-associated graft-versus-host disease (TA-GVHD). In this process, ionizing radiation is used to damage T cell DNA, thereby preventing donor T cell proliferation, engraftment, and subsequent TA-GVHD. As per *AABB* standards, the intended dose of irradiation should be at least 25 gray (Gy) (2500 cGy) but not more than 50 Gy, delivered to the central portion of the container. No part of the container can receive less than 15 Gy [65]. Of note, European standards require a higher dose with no area of the container receiving less than 25 Gy. Irradiation sources available in the United States include either cesium-137 (^{137}CS) or cobalt-60 (^{60}Co) with verification of dose delivery using a fully loaded canister either annually (cesium-137) or semiannually (cobalt-60).

During the radioactive decay process, high-energy photons are emitted that damage and inactivate T cell nucleic acids. Cellular products including red cells, platelets, nonfrozen (fresh) plasma, and granulocytes are treated with gamma irradiation. FFP and cryoprecipitate are considered acellular components and are not routinely irradiated. Irradiation of aliquots can be accomplished easily in blood centers for hospitals that have their own irradiator. Syringe sets can sometimes be difficult to irradiate as a maximally drawn plunger may not fit into the irradiator canister. This logistical problem can be solved by attaching and transferring the desired dose into a transfer pack than can be placed in the irradiator. After processing the blood or platelets can be redrawn back into the syringe and dispensed. Syringe aliquots can also be irradiated separately if they fit comfortably into the irradiator's canister [19, 46].

Indications

TA-GVHD is a rare but virtually universally fatal condition caused by the activation, proliferation, and engraftment of T lymphocytes. The pathogenesis of TA-GVHD requires certain criteria to be met before the host can be overtaken by donor lymphocytes. Firstly, the graft or donor product must contain viable T lymphocytes capable of mounting an immune response. Secondly, a recognizable disparity between host and donor HLA types must be present. Lastly, the recipient must be incapable of rejecting the immunocompetent donor cells [26]. The last requirement can be caused by either an immunocompromised state or by a shared HLA haplotype. A heterozygous recipient may not be able to recognize homozygous donor T cells as foreign. Unfortunately the donor T cells can be stimulated by the non-shared HLA antigen resulting in donor T cell expansion, dysregulated cytokine release, and overwhelming inflammatory response. This phenomenon can be seen when transfusing components from related donors into immunocompetent recipients [53, 68]. The same T cell activation process is initiated in an immunocompromised host who is unable to mount a response to foreign HLA antigens.

TA-GVHD most commonly manifests as gastrointestinal tract bleeding, erythematous macropapular skin eruption, progressive hepatic dysfunction, and hypoproliferative pancytopenia in a background of nonspecific symptoms such as fever, anorexia, nausea, and vomiting. The onset of symptoms typically occurs within 8–10 days after transfusion with a mortality rate of 89.7 % at a median of 24 days after exposure. The cause of death is attributed to profound bone marrow failure resulting in overwhelming infection or bleeding. Definitive diagnosis relies on both clinical findings and concurrent biopsy demonstrating lymphocyte infiltration into affected tissues or the persistence of donor lymphocytes in peripheral circulation [39, 101]. Currently the mainstay of treatment involves immunosuppression. It should be noted that LR alone has been shown to be inadequate in preventing TA-GVHD.

The vulnerability of the pediatric population has long been considered. Some of the first reported cases of TA-GVHD occurred in immunocompromised fetuses and infants [29, 61]. The clinical picture is similar to that seen in adults but may follow a different timeline with a median onset of symptoms occurring at 28 days and death at 51 days [64]. According to the *AABB* standards, cellular components must be irradiated if the patient is considered to be at risk for GVHD, if the patient is receiving a directed donation from a relative, or if the recipient is receiving HLA-compatible products. Many institutions have set standards to include a wider range of eligible patients. This is due to the difficulty sometimes in identifying neonates who are immunosuppressed and at risk for TA-GVHD. To address this concern, some institutions have elected to irradiate all products for all patients, while others have set institutional guidelines of requiring irradiation up to a certain neonatal age, for example, 1 or 4 months. The lack of clinical trials creates much variability in these guidelines and practices across pediatric hospitals. Table 1.3 highlights well-documented indications for the administration of irradiated products.

Unlike LR, irradiation has known deleterious effects on blood products. The half-life of red blood cells is limited to 28 days after the date of irradiation. In the United States, products can be irradiated at any point before their expiration date. The shortened shelf life is implemented due to the damaging effects of irradiation on red blood cell membranes and the resulting leakage of potassium, hemoglobin, and lactate dehydrogenase into the extracellular fluid. In addition, reduction in 2,3-DPG and ATP has also been observed [74, 104]. In a recent Australian study, irradiated red blood cells demonstrated significantly higher extracellular potassium levels

Table 1.3 Indications for the administration of irradiated products [19, 51]

Documented indications	Potential indications	Usually not indicated
Intrauterine transfusions	Other malignancies	Patients with human immunodeficiency virus
Premature neonates	Donor-recipient pairs from genetically homogenous population	Full-term infants
Low birth weight neonates		Immunocompetent patients
Known or suspected immune deficiency [72]		
Chemotherapy or radiation-related immunosuppression [72]		
Erythroblastosis fetalis in neonates		
Hematologic malignancies		
Solid tumors (neuroblastoma, sarcoma, Hodgkin's disease)		
Stem cell transplant		
Crossmatched components		
HLA-matched components		
Directed donations from family members		
Fludarabine therapy		
Granulocyte components		

Adapted from AABB Technical Manual, 18th Edition [51]

compared to controls just 2 h post irradiation. Additionally, red blood cells irradiated after 8–10 days of storage produced higher extracellular levels of potassium compared to fresher red blood cell units [98]. Similar findings have led to suggested revisions of North American guidelines regarding the use of red blood cell units that have been irradiated at later stages of storage [77]. Accelerated potassium leakage holds special importance for neonates, as this population is at risk to suffer from cardiotoxicity caused by transfusion-induced hyperkalemia. The Council of Europe for pediatric transfusion recommends transfusion within 48 h post irradiation [22]. While small-volume transfusions are not likely to cause cardiac arrhythmias due to dilution effects, neonates requiring large-volume transfusions or red cell exchange should receive red blood cells irradiated at issue or washed and resuspended in sterile saline [45, 46, 101]. Many institutions will either irradiate the blood just prior to transfusion of large volumes or rewash irradiated blood after several days to reduce the risk of hyperkalemic reactions. In contrast, platelets are unaffected by irradiation doses <50 Gy and remain stable for the length of their 5-day shelf life [93].

Fresh Products

RBCs stored at 1–6 °C gradually leak potassium into the supernatant plasma over time. In fresh units the potassium level is less than 5 mEq. At expiration, undisturbed RBC units can demonstrate potassium levels of 5–7 mEq [51]. The rate of leakage is determined by several factors including anticoagulant-preservative solution used and secondary processing such as irradiation. Products stored in AS-1, AS-3, and AS-5 have lower rates of potassium leakage compared to those stored in CPDA-1 [52, 84]. In the adult populations, increased potassium levels are rarely of consequence. Furthermore, small volume (10–15 ml/kg) administered slowly has been shown to have little effect in infants younger than 4 months old [75]. However, concern for hyperkalemia in premature infants and neonates receiving large-volume transfusions has long been debated [52]. Hyperkalemia in newborns is defined as a potassium level greater than 6 mmol/l. Elevated potassium levels affect myocyte membrane potential resulting in cardiac arrhythmias with small or premature infants who have had recent cardiac surgery of venous catheter placement at greatest risk [50]. Hyperkalemia warrants a medical emergency. For this reason, many blood banks have instituted policies requiring the release of "fresh" blood components less than 5–14 days old. Washing (discussed below) is sometimes reserved for older units.

Although newer blood units are often used for newborns, the true benefits of avoiding prolonged storage have not been clearly defined. Several studies in the adult population have associated the use of older blood units with reduced survival rates and increased complications. One retrospective study in adult patients undergoing cardiac surgery associated transfusion of blood units older than 2 weeks with higher mortality rates and increased adverse events including renal failure, sepsis multisystem organ failure, and the need for prolonged ventilatory support compared to patients who received fresher units [38]. Another observational study in critically ill adult patients in New Zealand and Australia demonstrated similar findings, linking exposure of older red blood cells with increased mortality [67]. It is hypothesized that the underlying mechanism of this association is at least in part due to the functional decline of red cells during storage. Unfortunately, the cause and effect relationship cannot be clearly delineated due to the intrinsic limitations of observational studies including uncontrollable confounding variables such as population heterogeneity and temporal changes during the study period [42]. In contrast to previous adult studies, a Canadian double-blind randomized controlled trial of 377 premature low birth weight infants (<1250 g) demonstrated that the use of fresh RBCs (<7 days old) did not improve outcomes. The transfusion of fresher RBCs showed no benefit or harm in regard to mortality, infection, or length of stay in the NICU [24]. These findings suggest that the age of red cells is perhaps not as important in the neonatal population as once thought. The inconsistent findings from prior studies have implications for blood bank inventory. Requests or policies requiring newer units pose logistical challenges in inventory management particularly in blood centers operating under a dedicated donor policy. Currently, there is no consensus regarding the required age of RBC units dispensed to neonates. Current policy is institution dependent.

Washing and Volume Reduction

Occasionally, requests for washed products are placed. RBCs and platelets can be washed using an automated system (preferred) or manually with 1–2 L of sterile normal saline. Washing is accomplished by using centrifugation to remove up to 98 % of plasma with resuspension of the remaining product in sterile saline [101]. Washing results in up to 20 % of RBC and 30 % of platelet loss. In addition, washing creates an open system. RBCs must be transfused within 24 h after washing. Platelets must be transfused within 4 h. Washing also results in red blood cell damage and increased potassium leak [101]. It is therefore prudent to transfuse RBCs within the first 12 h after washing.

Volume reduction is a similar process to washing where plasma and/or additive solution is partially removed from cellular blood components. The volume reduction of platelets is typically performed to reduce the amount of plasma for patients at risk for cardiac overload or for intrauterine infusions. Platelets from WB are volume reduced by centrifugation to 10–15 mL/unit. Platelet recovery rate is 85 % after volume reduction. Apheresis platelets can also be subject to volume reduction; however, previous study indicates that volume reduction can result in increased platelet activation and impaired aggregation [76] and is not necessary for routine transfusions.

Historically, washing of cellular components was performed commonly to remove WBCs before the advent of leukoreduction. In modern transfusion medicine, washing is performed to remove three substances: plasma, anticoagulant-preservative solutions, and potassium. In some instances, maternal cells must be washed before transfusion in the treatment of hemolytic disease of the newborn or neonatal alloimmune thrombocytopenia (NAIT). Washed RBCs are indicated in the following situations: (1) large-volume transfusion of older RBCs that have been irradiated >48 h before transfusion, (2) patients who experience recurrent severe transfusion reactions, (3) patients with IgA deficiency for whom IgA-deficient blood is not available, (4) patients at risk for hyperkalemia-induced cardiac arrhythmias, and (5) patients with alloimmune cytopenias receiving maternally derived blood components [20, 75, 101]. Washing can be used to reduce additive solution; however, this may not be necessary. On occasion, blood bank inventory may wane, limiting options to platelets that are ABO incompatible. In the adult setting, "out of type" platelets can be safely transfused; however, in neonates the incompatible antibodies present in the donor plasma can cause hemolysis [40]. Volume-reduced platelets may be indicated in this setting if the transfusion is urgent. In some pediatric hospitals, the anti-A titer is determined prior to transfusion. A high titer, defined as >1:64, is considered unsafe for transfusion without further modification.

References

1. AABB, ARC, ABC, ASBP. Circular of information for the use of human blood and blood components. 2013.
2. AABB. Information piece: alternatives to transfusable single-donor plasma components. 2014.
3. AABB, Clinical Transfusion Medicine Committee; Heddle NM, Boeckh M, Grossman B, Jacobson J, Kleinman S, Tobian AAR, Webert K, Wong ECC, Roback JD. AABB Committee Report: reducing transfusion-transmitted cytomegalovirus infections. Transfusion. 2016.
4. Abonnenc M, Sonego G, Kaiser-Guignard J, et al. *In vitro* evaluation of pathogen-inactivated buffy coat-derived platelet concentrates during storage: psoralen-based photochemical treatment step-by-step. Blood Transfus. 2015;13(2):255–64.
5. Bandarenko N, editor. Blood transfusion therapy: a physician's handbook. 11th ed. Bethesda: AABB; 2014.
6. Blajchman MA, Goldman M, Freedman JJ, Sher GD. Proceedings of a consensus conference: prevention of post-transfusion CMV in the era of universal leukoreduction. Transfus Med Rev. 2001;15:1–20.
7. Brecher ME, Means N, et al. Evaluation of automated of an automated culture system for detecting bacterial contamination of platelets: an analysis with 15 contaminating organisms. Transfusion. 2001;41:477–82.
8. Brugnara C, Platt OS. The neonatal erythrocyte and its disorders. In: Nathan DG, Orkin SH, editors. Nathan and Oskis hematology of infancy and childhood. 7th ed. Philadelphia: WB Saunders; 2009. p. 21–66.
9. Burghardt D. Component preparation and storage. In: Hillyer C, Strauss RG, Luban N, editors. Handbook of pediatric transfusion medicine. London: Elsevier; 2004. p. 11–25.
10. Callum JL, Karkouti K, Yulia L. Cryoprecipitate: the current state of knowledge. Transfus Med Rev. 2009;23:177–88.
11. Cancelas JA, Dumont LJ, Maes LA, Rugg N, Herschel L, Whitley PH, Szczepiokowski ZM, Siegel AH, Hess JR, Zia M. Additive solution-7 reduces the red blood cell cold storage lesion. Transfusion. 2015;55:491–8.
12. Ciavarella D, Snyder E. Clinical use of blood transfusion devices. Transfus Med Rev. 1988;2:95.

13. Cohn CS, Stubbs J, Schwartz J, Francis R, Goss C, Cushing M, Shaz B, Mair D, Brantigan B, Heaton WA. A comparison of adverse reaction rates for PAS C versus plasma platelet units. Transfusion. 2014;54:1927–34.
14. DePalma L. Red cell alloantibody formations in the neonate and infant: considerations for current immunohematologic practice. Immunohematology. 1992;8:33–7.
15. Diab YA, Wong ECC, Luban NLC. Massive transfusion in children and neonates. Br J Haematol. 2013;161:15–26.
16. Downes K, Shulman I. Pretransfusion testing. In: Fung M, Grossman BJ, Hillyer CD, Westhoff C, editors. Technical manual. 18th ed. Bethesda: AABB; 2014. p. 367–90.
17. Doyle JJ. The role of erythropoietin in anemia of prematurity. Semin Perinatol. 1997;21: 20–7.
18. Dumont LJ, Gulliksson H, van der Meer PF, et al. Interruption of agitation of platelet concentrates: a multicenter in vitro study by the BEST collaborative on the effects of shipping platelets. Transfusion. 2007;47:1666–73.
19. Dumont L, Papari M, Aronson C, Dumont D. Whole-blood collection and component processing. In: Fung M, Grossman BJ, Hillyer CD, Westhoff C, editors. Technical manual. 18th ed. Bethesda: AABB; 2014. p. 135–65.
20. Dunbar N. Hospital storage, monitoring, pretransfusion processing, distribution, and inventory management of blood components. In: Fung M, Grossman BJ, Hillyer CD, Westhoff C, editors. Technical manual. 18th ed. Bethesda: AABB; 2014. p. 213–29.
21. D'Alessandro A, Hansen KC, Silliman CC, Moore EE, Kelher M, Banerjee A. Metabolomics of AS-5 RBC supernatants following routine storage. Vox sanguinis. 2015;108(2):131–40.
22. European Committee (Partial Agreement) on Blood Transfusion (CD-PTS): Guide to the Preparation, Use and Quality Assurance of Blood Components. 14th ed. Strasbourg: Council of Europe; 2008.
23. Fergusson D, Hébert PC, Lee SK, Walker CR, Barrington KJ, Joseph L, Blajchman MA, Shapiro S. Clinical outcomes following institution of universal leukoreduction of blood transfusions for premature infants. JAMA. 2003;289(15):1950–6.
24. Fergusson DA, Hébert P, Hogan DL, LeBel L, Rouvinez-Bouali N, Smyth JA, Sankaran K, Tinmouth A, Blajchman MA, Kovacs L, Lachance C, Lee S, Walker CR, Hutton B, Ducharme R, Balchin K, Ramsay T, Ford JC, Kakadekar A, Ramesh K, Shapiro S. Effect of fresh red blood cell transfusions on clinical outcomes in premature, very low-birth-weight infants: the ARIPI randomized trial. JAMA. 2012;308(14):1443–51.
25. Galel S. Infectious disease screening. In: Fung M, Grossman BJ, Hillyer CD, Westhoff C, editors. Technical manual. 18th ed. Bethesda: AABB; 2014. p. 179–212.
26. Gokhale SG, Gokhale SS. Transfusion-associated graft versus host disease (TAGVHD)–with reference to neonatal period. J Matern Fetal Neonatal Med. 2015;28(6):700–4. Epub 2014 Jul 1.
27. Gruenwald CE, McCrindle BW, Crawford-Lean L, et al. Reconstituted fresh whole blood improves clinical outcomes compared with stored component blood therapy for neonates undergoing cardiopulmonary bypass for cardiac surgery: a randomized controlled trial. J Thorac Cardiovasc Surg. 2008;136(6):1442–9.
28. Gulliksson H. Platelets from platelet-rich-plasma versus buffy-coat-derived platelets: what is the difference? Revista Brasileira de Hematologia e Hemoterapia. 2012;34(2):76–7.
29. Hathaway WE, Githens JH, Blackburn WR, Fulginiti V, Kempe CH. Aplastic anemia, histiocytosis and erythroderma in immunologically deficient children. Probable human runt disease. N Engl J Med. 1965;273(18):953–8.
30. Hiroshi A, Junichi H, Mitsuaki A, Hisami I. Platelet additive solution: electrolytes. Transfus Apher Sci. 2011;44(3):277–81.
31. Ho M. Epidemiology of cytomegalovirus infections. Rev Inf Dis. 1990;12 Suppl 7:S701–10.
32. Högman CF, Knutson F, Lööf H. Storage of whole blood before separation: the effect of temperature on red cell 2,3 DPG and the accumulation of lactate. Transfusion. 1999;39(5):492–7.
33. Jain R, Jarosz C. Safety and efficacy of AS-1 red blood cell use in neonates. Transfus Apher Sci. 2001;24:111–5.

34. Jobes DR, Sesok-Pizzini D, Friedman D. Reduced Transfusion Requirement With Use of Fresh Whole Blood in Pediatric Cardiac Surgical Procedures. Ann Thorac Surg. 2015; 99:1706–12.

35. Josephson CD, Caliendo AM, Easley KA, et al. Blood transfusion and breast milk transmission of cytomegalovirus in very low-birth-weight infants: a prospective cohort study. JAMA Pediatr. 2014;168(11):1054–62.

36. Josephson C, Meyer J. Neonatal and pediatric transfusion practice. In: Fung M, Grossman BJ, Hillyer CD, Westhoff C, editors. Technical manual. 18th ed. Bethesda: AABB; 2014. p. 571–97.

37. Klein HG, Dodd RY, et al. Current status of microbial contamination of blood components: summary of a conference. Transfusion. 1997;37:95–101.

38. Koch CG, Li L, Sessler DI, Figueroa P, Hoeltge GA, Mihaljevic T, Blackstone EH. Duration of red-cell storage and complications after cardiac surgery. N Engl J Med. 2008;358(12): 1229–39.

39. Kopolovic I, Ostro J, Tsubota H, et al. A systematic review of transfusion-associated graft-versus-host disease. Blood. 2015;126(3):406–14.

40. Larsson LG, Welsh VJ, Ladd DJ. Acute intravascular hemolysis secondary to out of group platelet transfusion. Transfusion. 2000;40:902–6.

41. Lee D, Slagle T, Jackson T, Evans C. Reducing blood donor exposures in low birth weight infants by the use of older, unwashed packed red blood cells. J Pediatr. 1995;126(2):280–6.

42. Lelubre C, Piagnerelli M, Vincent JL. Association between duration of storage of transfused red blood cells and morbidity and mortality in adult patients: myth or reality? Transfusion. 2009;49:1384–94.

43. Lin L, Dikeman R, Molini B, Lukehart SA, Lane R, Dupuis K, Metzel P, Corash L. Photochemical treatment of platelet concentrates with amotosalen and long-wavelength ultraviolet light inactivates a broad spectrum of pathogenic bacteria. Transfusion. 2004;44:1496–504.

44. Liu E, Mannino F, Lane T. Prospective, randomized trial of the safety and efficacy of a limited donor exposure transfusion program for premature neonates. J Pediatr. 1994;125(1):92–6.

45. Luban NLC, Strauss RG, Hume HA. Commentary on the safety of red blood cells preserved in extended storage media for neonatal transfusions. Transfusion. 1991;31:229–35.

46. Luban NLC. Irradiation for neonatal and pediatric transfusion. In: Herman J, Manno C, editors. Pediatric transfusion therapy. Bethesda: AABB; 2002. p. 147–69.

47. Ludvigsen C, Swanson JL, Thompson TR, McCullogh J. The failure of neonates to form red cell alloantibodies in response to multiple transfusions. Am J Clin Pathol. 1987;87:250–1.

48. Mangel J, Goldman M, Garcia C, Spurll G. Reduction of donor exposures in premature infants by the use of designated adenine-saline preserved split red blood cell packs. J Perinatol. 2001;21(6):363–7.

49. Manno CS, Hedberg KW, Kim HC, Bunin GR, Nicolson S, Jobes D, Schwartz E, Norwood WI. Comparison of the hemostatic effects of fresh whole blood, stored whole blood and components after open heart surgery in children. Blood. 1991;77(5):930–6.

50. Masilamani K, van der Voort J. The management of acute hyperkalaemia in neonates and children. Arch Dis Child. 2012;97(4):376–80. doi:10.1136/archdischild-2011-300623. Epub 2011 Sep 13.

51. Mazzei C, Papovsky M, Kopko P. Noninfectious Complications of Blood Transfusion. In: Fung M, Grossman BJ, Hillyer CD, Westhoff C, editors. Technical Manual. 18th edition. Bethesda: AABB; 2014. p. 665–96.

52. McDonald TB, Berkowitz RA. Massive transfusion in children. In: Jeffries LC, Brecher ME, editors. Massive transfusion. Bethesda: AABB; 1994. p. 97–119.

53. McMilan KD, Johnson RL. HLA-homozygosity and the risk of related-donor transfusion-associated graft versus host disease. Transfus Med Rev. 1993;7:37–41.

54. Mendrone A, Fabrone A, Langhi D, et al. Is there justification for universal leukoreduction? Rev Bras Hematol Hemoter. 2014;36(4):237.

55. Metcalfe P, Williamson LM, Reutelingsperger CP, Swann I, Ouwehand WH, Goodall AH. Activation during storage of therapeutic platelets affects deterioration during storage: a

comparative flow cytometric study of different production methods. Br J Haematol. 1997; 98(1):86–95.

56. Mohan P, Brocklehurst P. Granulocyte transfusions for neonates with confirmed or suspected sepsis and neutropaenia. Cochrane Database Syst Rev. 2003:CD003956.

57. Mok YH, Lee JH, Cheifetz IM. Neonatal extracorporeal membrane oxygenation: update on management strategies and long-term outcomes. Adv Neonatal Care. 2016;16(1):26–36.

58. Moroff G, Holme S, George VM, Heaton WA. Effect on platelet properties of exposure to temperatures below 20 degrees C for short periods during storage at 20 to 24 degrees C. Transfusion. 1994;34(4):317–21.

59. Mou S, Giroir B, Molitor-Kirsch E. Fresh whole blood versus reconstituted blood for pump priming in heart surgery in infants. N Engl J Med. 2004;351:1635–44.

60. Murphy K, O'Brien P, O'Donnell J. Acquired protein s deficiency in thrombotic thrombocytopenic purpura patients receiving solvent/detergent plasma exchange. Br J Haematol. 2003;122:518–9.

61. Naiman JL, Punnett HH, Lischner HW, Destine ML, Arey JB. Possible graft-versus-host reaction after intrauterine transfusion for Rh erythroblastosis fetalis. N Engl J Med. 1969;281(13):697–701.

62. Nance ST, Meny G. Compatibility issues in neonatal and pediatric transfusion. In: Herman J, Manno C, editors. Pediatric transfusion therapy. Bethesda: AABB; 2002.

63. Nomani AZ, Nabi Z, Rashid H, Janjua J, Nomani H, Majeed A, Chaudry SR, Mazhar AS. Osmotic nephrosis with mannitol: review article. Ren Fail. 2014;36(7):1169–76. Epub 2014 Jun 18.

64. Ohto H, Anderson KC. Posttransfusion graft-versus-host disease in Japanese newborns. Transfusion. 1996;36(2):117–23. Review.

65. Ooley P, editor. Standards for blood banks and transfusion services. 30th ed. Bethesda: AABB, 2016.

66. Pietersz RN, deKorte D, Reesink HW, et al. Storage of whole blood for up to 24 hours at ambient temperature prior to component preparation. Vox Sang. 1989;56:145–50.

67. Pettilä V, Westbrook AJ, Nichol AD, Bailey MJ, Wood EM, Syres G, Phillips LE, Street A, French C, Murray L, Orford N, Santamaria JD, Bellomo R, Cooper DJ, Blood Observational Study Investigators for ANZICS Clinical Trials Group. Age of red blood cells and mortality in the critically ill. Crit Care. 2011;15(2):R116. Epub 2011 Apr 15.

68. Petz LD, Calhoun L, Yam P, et al. Transfusion associated graft-versus-host disease in immunocompetent patients. Report of a fatal case associated with transfusion of blood from a second degree relative, and a survey of predisposing factors. Transfusion. 1993;33:742–50.

69. Roback J. Preparation of blood components to reduce cytomegalovirus and other infectious risks. In: Hillyer C, Strauss RG, Luban N, editors. Handbook of pediatric transfusion medicine. London: Elsevier; 2004. p. 93–9.

70. Roback JD, Bray RA, Hillyer CD. Longitudinal monitoring of WBC subsets in packed RBC units after filtration: implications for transfusion transmission of infections. Transfusion. 2000;40:500–6.

71. Rock G, Poon A, Haddad S, Romans R, St Louis P. Nutricel as an additive solution for neonatal transfusion. Transf Sci. 1999;20:29–36.

72. Roseff SD, Luban NL, Manno CS. Guidelines for assessing appropriateness of pediatric transfusion. Transfusion. 2002;42:1398–413.

73. Roseff SD. Pediatric blood collection and transfusion technology. In Herman JK, Manno CS, eds. Pediatric Transfusion Therapy. Bethesda, MD: AABB Press; 2002:217–47.

74. Samuel LH, Anderson G, Mintz PD. Rejuvenation of irradiated AS-1 red cells. Transfusion. 1997;37:25–8.

75. Sandler S, Ramasethu J. Washed and/or volume-reduced blood components. In: Hillyer C, Strauss RG, Luban N, editors. Handbook of pediatric transfusion medicine. London: Elsevier; 2004. p. 113–20.

76. Schoenfield H, Muhm M, Doepfmer UR, et al. The functional integrity in volume reduced platelet concentrates. Anesth Analg. 2005;100:78–81.

77. Serrano K, Chen D, Hansen AL, et al. The effect of timing of gamma-irradiation on hemolysis and potassium release in leukoreduced red cell con- © 2014 International Society of Blood Transfusion Vox Sanguinis (2015) 108, 141–150 Effect of irradiation on K+ levels 149 concentrates stored in SAGM. Vox Sang. 2014;106:379–81.

78. Simone ER. Adenine and blood banking. Transfusion. 1977;17:317–25.

79. Smith D, Lu Q, Yuan S, Goldfinger D, Fernando LP, Ziman A. Survey of current practice for prevention of transfusion-transmitted cytomegalovirus in the United States: leucoreduction vs. cytomegalovirus-seronegative. Vox Sang. 2010;98:29–36.

80. Smith SW. Blood Component Collection by Apheresis. In: Fung M, Grossman BJ, Hillyer CD, Westhoff C, eds. Technical Manual. 18th edition. Bethesda: AABB; 2014. p.167–78.

81. Snyder EL, Hezzey A, Katz AJ, Bock J. Occurrence of the release reaction during preparation and storage of platelet concentrates. Vox Sang. 1981;41(3):172–7.

82. Strauss RG, Burmeister LF, Johnson K, James T, Miller J, Cordle DG, Bell EF, Ludwig GA. AS-1 red cells for neonatal transfusions: a randomized trial assessing donor exposure and safety. Transfusion. 1996;36(10):873–8.

83. Strauss RG, Burmeister LF, Johnson K, Cress G, Cordle D. Feasibility and safety of AS-3 red blood cells for neonatal transfusions. J Pediatr. 2000;136(2):215–9.

84. Strauss RG. Data driven blood banking practices for neonatal RBC transfusions. Transfusion. 2000;40(12):1528–40.

85. Strauss RG. Additive solutions and product age in neonatal red blood cell transfusion. In: Herman J, Manno C, editors. Pediatric transfusion therapy. Bethesda: AABB; 2002. p. 129–45.

86. Stroncek D. Neonatal alloimmune neutropenia and alloimmune thrombocytopenia. In: Herman J, Manno C, editors. Pediatric transfusion therapy. Bethesda: AABB; 2002. p. 109–27.

87. Tobian AAR, Fuller AK, Uglik K, et al. The impact of platelet additive solution apheresis platelets on allergic transfusion reactions and corrected count increment. Transfusion. 2014;54(6):1523–9.

88. Tuchschmid P, Mieth D, Burger R, Duc G. Potential hazard of hypoalbuminemia in newborn babies after exchange transfusions with ADSOL red blood cell concentrates. Pediatrics. 1990;85(2):234–5.

89. U.S. Food and Drug Administration/Center for Drug Evaluation and Research. Guidance for industry: barcode label requirements questions and answers. Silver Springs, 2011.

90. U.S. Food and Drug Administration/Dept of Health and Human Services. Approval letter. Octaplas. 2013.

91. U. S. Food and Drug Administration. Summary of safety and effectiveness data: INTERCEPT blood system for platelets. 2014.

92. van Rossum H, de Kraa N, Thomas M, Holleboom C, Castel A, van Rossum A. Comparison of the direct antiglobulin test and the eluate technique for diagnosing haemolytic disease of the newborn. Pract Lab Med. 2015;3:17–22.

93. Voak D, Chapman J, Finney RD, et al. Guidelines to gamma irradiation of blood components for the prevention of transfusion associated graft versus host disease. Trans Med. 1996;261–71.

94. Walker P, Hamilton J. Identification of antibodies to red cell antigens. In: Fung M, Grossman BJ, Hillyer CD, Westhoff C, editors. Technical manual. 18th ed. Bethesda: AABB; 2014. p. 391–424.

95. Walsh S, Murphy J. Neonatal jaundice—are we over-treating? Iran Med J. 2010;103(1):28–9.

96. Wang-Rodriguez J, Fry E, Fiebig E, Lee T, Busch M, Mannino F, Lane TA. Immune response to blood transfusion in very-low-birthweight infants. Transfusion. 2000;40(1):25–34.

97. Wang-Rodriguez J. The fetal/neonatal immune response. In: Herman J, Manno C, editors. Pediatric transfusion therapy. Bethesda: AABB; 2002. p. 1–23.

98. Winter K, Johnson L, Kwok M, et al. Understanding the effects of gamma-irradiation on potassium levels in red cell concentrates stored in SAG-M for neonatal red cell transfusion. Vox Sang. 2015;108:141–50.

99. Wollowitz S. Fundamentals of the psoralen-based Helinx technology for inactivation of infectious pathogens and leukocytes in platelets and plasma. Semin Hematol. 2001;38 Suppl 11:4–11.
100. Wong E, Roseff SD, editors. Pediatric hemotherapy data card. Bethesda: AABB; 2009.
101. Wong E, Josephson C, Punzalan R, Roseff S, Sesok-Pizzini D, Sloan S, Strauss R, editors. Pediatric transfusion: a physician's handbook. Bethesda: AABB; 2015.
102. Yarraton H, Lawrie AS, Mackie IJ, et al. Coagulation factor levels in cryosupernatant prepared from plasma treated with amotosalen hydrochloride (S-59) and ultraviolet A light. Transfusion. 2005;45:1453–8.
103. Wu Y, Zou S, Cable R, Dorsey K, Tang Y, Hapip CA, Melmed R, Trouern-Trend J, Wang J-H, Champion M, Fang C, Dodd R. Direct assessment of cytomegalovirus transfusion-transmitted risks after universal leukoreduction. Transfusion. 2010;50:776–86.
104. Zimmermann R, Wintzheimer S, Weisbach V, et al. Influence of prestorage leukoreduction and subsequent irradiation on in vitro red blood cell storage variables of red blood cells in additive solution saline-adenine-glucose-mannitol. Transfusion. 2009;49:75–80.

Chapter 2
Blood Product Administration

Grace Hsu and Paul A. Stricker

Neonates are a patient population with special considerations in relation to blood transfusion. Preterm neonates, particularly extremely low birth weight (ELBW, birth weight <1000 g) and very low birth weight (VLBW, birth weight <1500 g), and critically ill neonates are among the most frequently transfused patient groups – with the volume of blood transfused inversely related to the weight and gestational age of the baby [1]. Because of advances in neonatal intensive care, including advances in blood component administration [2], smaller and more premature infants are surviving. This chapter discusses blood components and their suggested indications for transfusion in neonates and reviews vascular access, blood product filters, and warmers. This chapter also presents the use of antifibrinolytics and perioperative transfusion monitoring in neonates.

Neonatal Size and Blood Volumes

A full-term neonate has a circulating blood volume of 80–90 mL/kg. Preterm and low-birth-weight neonates have a higher circulating blood volume (90–100 mL/kg). There is some variability, especially in the immediate neonatal period, with higher blood volumes seen in premature neonates in whom cord clamping is delayed or when cord milking is performed during delivery. This practice has been shown to increase both hematocrit and blood volume [3]. In 2012, a Cochrane review compared immediate cord clamping versus delayed cord clamping. The results of this review suggested that delaying cord clamping for 30–120 s was associated with less

G. Hsu, MD (✉) • P.A. Stricker, MD
Department of Anesthesiology and Critical Care Medicine, Perelman School of Medicine
University of Pennsylvania, The Children's Hospital of Philadelphia, 3401 Civic Center
Boulevard, Philadelphia, PA 19104, USA
e-mail: hsug@email.chop.edu; strickerp@email.chop.edu

© Springer International Publishing Switzerland 2017   29
D.A. Sesok-Pizzini (ed.), *Neonatal Transfusion Practices*,
DOI 10.1007/978-3-319-42764-5_2

need for transfusion, less intraventricular hemorrhage (IVH), and lower risk for necrotizing enterocolitis in preterm neonates [4].

Blood Components, Indications for Transfusion, and Transfusion Dosing

Neonatal transfusion is an ever-evolving area of practice that until fairly recently was largely not evidence based and mostly adapted from pediatric and adult practices [5]. Evidence to guide neonatal transfusion decision-making has grown considerably, yet in many circumstances, there remains no consensus for triggers and indications for blood product administration in our smallest patients [6, 7], and consequently, transfusion practices remain widely variable [8–10]. The following sections present the current state of evolving guidelines for blood component transfusion in neonates.

Packed Red Blood Cells

Red blood cells (RBCs) are transfused to increase oxygen-carrying capacity and optimize tissue oxygen delivery. Packed red blood cells (PRBCs) are the most commonly available blood component with RBCs. When deciding to transfuse PRBCs, it is important that the clinician take into consideration a patient's clinical status and whether clinical symptoms of anemia are present. Signs of anemia in a neonate may include tachycardia, tachypnea, dyspnea, apneic episodes, decreased urine output, and lethargy. Thresholds for transfusion vary according to the clinical scenario and are different for a healthy full-term baby, a premature neonate with chronic lung disease, and a neonate with cyanotic congenital heart disease.

A full-term infant who is otherwise healthy may tolerate a hemoglobin level as low as 7 g/dL without any symptoms of anemia or inadequate tissue oxygen delivery. However, an acutely ill neonate (e.g., sepsis, necrotizing enterocolitis) requiring oxygen therapy or ventilatory support may require higher hemoglobin levels to produce higher oxygen-carrying capacity and oxygen delivery, which may in turn reduce cardiac and respiratory work, and prevent apnea. Guidelines have been published for PRBC transfusion in full-term infants less than 4 months of age and are shown in Table 2.1 [6].

Neonates with uncorrected congenital cyanotic heart disease also require higher hemoglobin levels for adequate oxygen delivery. In these children, arterial blood is not fully saturated, and although the carrying capacity of the blood is normal, due to anatomic shunting, the effective oxygen-carrying capacity is markedly reduced. As a result, the critical hemoglobin concentration for adequate tissue oxygen delivery is higher. In these patients at rest, myocardial cells are functioning near the maximum

Table 2.1 Guidelines for transfusion of RBCs in full-term infants <4 months of age

1. Hematocrit <20 % with low reticulocyte count and symptoms of anemia:[a]
2. Hematocrit <30 % with an infant:
On <35 % hood O_2
On O_2 by nasal cannula
On continuous positive airway pressure (CPAP)/intermittent mandatory ventilation (IMV) with mechanical ventilation with mean airway pressure <6 cm H_2O
Significant apnea or bradycardia[b]
Significant tachycardia or tachypnea[c]
Low weight gain[d]
3. Hematocrit <35 % with an infant:
On >35 % hood O_2
On CPAP/IMV with mean airway pressure ≥6–8 cm H_2O
4. Hematocrit <45 % with an infant:
On ECMO
Congenital cyanotic heart disease

[a]Tachycardia, tachypnea, and poor feeding
[b]More than six episodes in 12 h or two episodes in 24 h requiring bag and mask ventilation while receiving therapeutic doses of methylxanthines
[c]Heart rate >180 beats/min for 24 h; respiratory rate >80 breaths/min for 24 h
[d]Gain of <10 g/day observed over 4 days while receiving ≥100 kcal/kg/day

oxygen extraction rate. During cardiac surgery, the myocytes are further strained, as ventricular function is impaired. However, there is little data to determine a specific threshold for transfusion in this patient population. Current recommendations are to transfuse to maintain hemoglobin greater than 15 g/dL [11, 12].

Preterm neonates are at high risk for anemia, because of frequent phlebotomies for laboratory testing, decreased endogenous erythropoietin production, lower hemoglobin at birth, and comorbid conditions. Adult clinical trials have shown restrictive transfusion strategies to be superior to liberal transfusion strategies, with decreased 30-day mortality, rates of cardiac complications, and rates of organ dysfunction in patients treated according to a restrictive transfusion strategy [13]. However, randomized trials in preterm neonates comparing low versus high hemoglobin transfusion thresholds have shown mixed outcomes. In one study, Bell et al. assigned 100 preterm ELBW and VLBW neonates to a restrictive or liberal transfusion arm. Thresholds were made depending on the age and respiratory status of the neonate. In the restrictive transfusion group, the hematocrit of infants was maintained at 22 % if not requiring positive pressure ventilation (PPV) or oxygen, 28 % if receiving nasal continuous positive airway pressure (CPAP) or oxygen, and 34 % if mechanically ventilated. This was compared to the liberal transfusion group, where the hematocrit was maintained at 30 % if not receiving PPV or oxygen, 38 % if on nasal CPAP or oxygen, and 46 % if mechanically ventilated. Patients in the restrictive arm were more likely to have intraparenchymal cerebral hemorrhage and periventricular leukomalacia. As expected, infants in the liberal transfusion group received more RBC transfusions. There were no differences in blood donor

Table 2.2 Hemoglobin threshold levels (g/dL) triggering RBC transfusion

		Low threshold		High threshold	
Age in days	Blood sampling	Respiratory support	No respiratory support	Respiratory support	No respiratory support
1–7	Capillary	≤11.5	≤10.0	≤13.5	≤12.0
	Central	≤10.4	≤9.0	≤12.2	≤10.9
8–14	Capillary	≤10.0	≤8.5	≤12.0	≤10.0
	Central	≤9.0	≤7.7	≤10.9	≤9.0
≥15	Capillary	≤8.5	≤7.5	≤10.0	≤8.5
	Central	≤7.7	≤6.8	≤9.0	≤7.7

exposures or percentage of infants who avoided transfusion altogether. The authors concluded that a restrictive transfusion practice may be harmful to premature infants, particularly in terms of their neurologic outcome [14].

In a second large trial, the Premature Infants in Need of Transfusion (PINT) study by Kirpalani et al., 451 ELBW infants were assigned to either a low or high hemoglobin transfusion threshold – with thresholds developed based on patient's age and requirement of respiratory support. Infants in the low hemoglobin threshold group had hemoglobin levels maintained from 6.8 to 11.5 g/dL. Neonates in the high hemoglobin threshold arm had hemoglobin levels maintained from 7.7 to 13.5 g/dL (Table 2.2). They compared mortality prior to discharge home and presence of retinopathy, bronchopulmonary dysplasia, or brain injury. Fewer infants in the low hemoglobin threshold group received one or more transfusions, and there were no differences between groups in all outcomes. The authors concluded that maintaining higher hemoglobin thresholds in ELBW infants had no additional benefit over low hemoglobin thresholds [15].

Based on these two studies, it is unclear what effect a low versus high hemoglobin threshold has on neurologic outcome in low-birth-weight infants. In a Cochrane review in 2011, Whyte and Kirpalani reviewed five trials comparing low versus high hemoglobin thresholds in preterm infants and recommended that clinicians not use higher levels of hemoglobin than used in these trials, to prevent over-transfusion, but to not go below the lower limits in these trials because of the potential risks of anemia [16].

Once a decision has been made to transfuse PRBCs and a target hemoglobin or hematocrit has been selected, the following "rules of thumb" can be used to determine the volume to be administered. Transfusion of 10–15 mL/kg of PRBCs will increase hemoglobin levels 1–2 g/dL. One can also calculate the volume of PRBCs to be transfused with the following equation [17]:

$$\text{Volume of PRBCs} = \frac{(\text{Desired Hct} - \text{Present Hct}) \times \text{Estimated Blood Volume}}{\text{Hematocrit of PRBCs}}$$

The hematocrit of a unit of PRBCs is around 60%, depending on the preservative used.

PRBCs are generally transfused over 1–2 h and are not to be at room temperature (20–24 °C) for longer than 4 h and, thus, need to be transfused within that time [18]. Intraoperative transfusion for acute blood loss may require faster administration rates.

Whole Blood

Transfusion of whole blood represented nearly all transfusion until the development of fractionation techniques and widespread adoption of component therapy. While the use of fractionated blood components has allowed for improved resource utilization and therapy targeted to specific patient needs, circumstances remain in which whole blood has advantages over individual component therapy. In adult patients, the principal modern application of whole blood transfusion is in the setting of massive transfusion secondary to traumatic injury (where massive transfusion is defined as replacement of a volume of blood that exceeds the circulating blood volume), with most reports originating from military experience in austere combat environments [19, 20].

From a mechanistic perspective, the advantage of replacement of massive blood loss with whole blood is that whole blood provides all components of coagulation (platelets, soluble clotting factors, RBCs) in addition to other plasma proteins that may be of physiologic importance. Furthermore, the operational complexities of coordinating the thawing and administration of multiple components are eliminated with whole blood administration. In the Vietnam conflict, Miller found that in previously healthy soldiers with major trauma and massive hemorrhage, coagulopathy did not develop in any soldier transfused less than 18 units of whole blood [21]. More recent investigations have demonstrated improved outcomes with "fresh" whole blood and warm fresh whole blood (from so-called walking blood banks) [22]. Whole blood with brief cold storage time may also have the advantage of minimized deleterious effects associated with prolonged storage on cellular components [23].

Although neonates rarely experience massive hemorrhage, circumstances exist in which whole blood has advantages over component therapy. These are in the setting of massive hemorrhage and transfusion and in the setting of neonatal cardiac surgery on cardiopulmonary bypass.

In particular, neonates undergoing cardiothoracic surgery with cardiopulmonary bypass (CPB) represent a patient group with predictable and significant transfusion requirements of multiple blood products. The volume of the CPB circuit can exceed the blood volume of a neonate. In infants and younger children, red blood cells must be included in pump primes to ensure an adequate hematocrit for tissue oxygen delivery when CPB is initiated. In neonates, priming of the CPB circuit with PRBCs and crystalloid and/or colloid results in profound dilution of soluble coagulation factors and platelets. This coupled with the lower normal circulating plasma concentrations of clotting proteins in neonates makes it necessary for CPB circuit primes to include red cells, clotting factors, and platelets to avoid significant dilutional coagulopathy upon initiation of CPB. The use of whole blood in bypass circuit primes allows for all necessary factors to be provided with a single blood donor exposure. Additionally, it has been demonstrated that this can be achieved with a split whole blood unit, where the other half is saved for transfusion following discontinuation of bypass or in the postoperative period as needed. With this approach, many neonates may only require a single blood donor exposure in the perioperative period [24]. This is significant in this population, as multiple blood donor exposures can increase the likelihood of alloimmunization, which is undesirable, as some of these children may need cardiac transplantation later in life.

Although massive hemorrhage and transfusion in neonates is rare outside of cardiac surgery, neonates undergoing tumor resections (e.g., sacrococcygeal teratoma resection) may benefit from fresh whole blood for replacement of losses to limit the potassium load. This remains relatively unstudied due to the unpredictable nature and relative rarity of these scenarios.

Reconstituted Blood

In part due to limited availability of whole blood, investigators have explored using reconstituted blood, which is composed of PRBCs and fresh frozen plasma (FFP) with or without platelets in the setting of neonatal cardiopulmonary bypass [25, 26]. One drawback of this approach is that transfusion of reconstituted blood made with PRBCs, FFP, and platelets results in three blood donor exposures compared to one that would be incurred with whole blood. In a study comparing fresh whole blood with reconstituted blood for CPB pump priming in infants, fresh whole blood did not have demonstrable advantages over reconstituted blood composed of PRBCs and FFP [25]. One subsequent study found reconstituted fresh whole blood was associated with improved outcomes (including clinical bleeding assessment, blood unit exposures, and reduced chest tube output) [26]. The use of reconstituted blood composed of PRBCs and FFP originating from the same donor has been applied in infants undergoing complex cranial vault reconstructive surgery. In this population of older infants, this donor-matched reconstituted blood resulted in near elimination of coagulopathy from dilution of soluble clotting factors, together with a reduction in blood donor exposures [27].

Fresh Frozen Plasma

Since the development of fractionation of blood products by Edward Cohn in the 1940s, FFP has been available for transfusion. FFP became more readily available in the 1960s when plasmapheresis was introduced as a way to collect plasma for fractionation [28]. Plasma is derived from whole blood and separated by centrifugation. When frozen within 8 h, the product is called FFP. FFP provides all coagulation factors, including the labile clotting factors V and VIII.

Previously, FFP has been used in the neonatal population in many clinical scenarios, including for volume expansion, correction of abnormal coagulation tests, and blood replacement in massive hemorrhage, although many of these practices do not have evidence to support their use. Recent guidelines have recommended more restricted indications for the use of FFP in neonates [29–31]. FFP transfusion is no longer recommended for volume replacement in neonates born less than 32 weeks gestation – as this practice has not been shown to decrease the incidence of death or to improve long-term neurologic outcome [32]. Additionally, FFP transfusion to prophylactically correct screening coagulation laboratory abnormalities is another practice that is no longer recommended [2]. Abnormal coagulation values in neonates, particularly in preterm infants, do not predict clinical bleeding [33].

Indications for FFP transfusion include [6, 29]:

1. Coagulopathy from multiple factor deficiencies, when prothrombin time (PT) > 1.5 × age-related normal value and partial thromboplastin time (PTT) > 1.5 × age-related normal value in a bleeding patient or one about to undergo an invasive procedure
2. Treatment of congenital deficiencies of single clotting factors when a specific factor concentrate is not available
3. In the treatment of disseminated intravascular coagulation (DIC)
4. Reversal of warfarin in an emergency situation, such as before an invasive procedure with active bleeding

FFP is stored at −18 °C or below. Prior to the administration of FFP, it must first be thawed at 37 °C for 30 min. It is then administered within 24 h if stored at 1–6 °C as after 6 h at this temperature, labile factors V and VIII begin to diminish [17]. If the thawed FFP is not transfused within 24 h, it is called thawed plasma (TP) and can be stored at 1–6 °C for another 4 days. While some clotting factors diminish during this time, they still remain within normal range [34, 35]. A dose of 10–15 mL/kg of FFP will raise plasma coagulation factor levels by 15–20 %. This effect lasts 6–12 h, so transfusion should be timed to clinical need, particularly for factor replacement prior to surgery and other invasive procedures [18].

As citrate anticoagulant is present in plasma, rapid administration of FFP (>1 mL/kg/min) is more frequently associated with citrate toxicity than with other blood components with smaller volumes of plasma, such as PRBCs. The rapid administration of FFP is particularly easy in neonates given their small size. Clinically, rapid FFP administration most commonly occurs in the treatment of hemorrhage; citrate toxicity manifests as myocardial depression, hypotension, and coagulation derangement. Additionally, neonates may be more susceptible to developing citrate toxicity, as the first-pass effect of the elimination of citrate via the liver is decreased in the first months of life [17].

Platelets

Thrombocytopenia or a platelet count of less than 150,000/μL is extremely common in the neonatal population, affecting close to a quarter of all infants admitted to the neonatal intensive care unit (NICU) and three-quarter of all ELBW infants [36]. Platelet transfusion is the only treatment for thrombocytopenia. Neonatal platelet transfusion practices vary widely in North America [37], and even more so world-wide [38], likely due in part to a lack of evidence to guide clinical practice. In the United States, a majority of platelet transfusions in neonates are prophylactic in those with no signs of clinical bleeding and with platelet counts greater than 50,000/μL [37, 39].

IVH is the most common form of major hemorrhage in preterm neonates and is a leading cause of morbidity and mortality in this patient group. Premature infants have underdeveloped subependymal matrices, along with other complex comorbidities, including cardiovascular instability and vascular fragility – which place them at risk of developing IVH. While thrombocytopenia has been associated with IVH [40], severity of thrombocytopenia does not necessarily correlate with risk of developing IVH. The strongest predictors of bleeding are gestational age less than 28 weeks, age less than 10 days old, and presence of necrotizing enterocolitis [41].

There is a paucity of high-level evidence to guide clinicians in determining the optimal threshold for platelet transfusion in neonates. There has only been one randomized, controlled trial in preterm neonates. In 1993, Andrew et al. randomized 152 ELBW and VLBW infants to either a treatment group where they transfused platelets to keep the platelet count greater than 150,000/μL or a control group where they transfused platelets to maintain the platelet count above 50,000/μL. This investigation revealed no difference in incidence or severity of IVH in the two groups (28 % in treatment group, 26 % in control group) [42].

Platelets are not only essential for maintenance of an intact endothelial barrier to prevent spontaneous hemorrhage but are also required for hemostasis with vascular injury during surgery. Given these considerations, Table 2.3 lists the recommendations for transfusing platelets in neonates [43].

Platelets are not usually indicated when thrombocytopenia is caused by destruction of autologous platelets (idiopathic thrombocytopenic purpura, heparin-induced thrombocytopenia, or thrombotic thrombocytopenic purpura) unless the patient is having a life-threatening hemorrhage.

Platelets are obtained by two different mechanisms. One process entails centrifugation of whole blood and yields at least 5.5×10 [10] platelets in 50–70 mLs of plasma from each unit of whole blood. One unit of whole blood-derived (WBD) platelets can be pooled with four to six other units to form one "dose" for an adult. One unit of WBD platelets is sufficient for a neonate. The second process for obtaining platelets is via apheresis, in which an apheresis machine extracts platelets from a donor's blood and then returns remaining blood back to the donor. A unit of apheresis-derived platelets contains greater than 3.0×10 [11] platelets in about 200 mLs of plasma. Platelets are stored at room temperature (20–24 °C). Because they

Table 2.3 Recommended platelet transfusion levels for neonates

Platelet count (×10⁹/L)	Guidelines
<30	Transfuse all
30–49	Transfuse if:
	Birth weight <1500 g and ≤7 days old
	Clinically unstable
	Concurrent coagulopathy
	Previous significant hemorrhage (i.e., grade 3 or 4 IVH)
	Prior to surgical procedure
	Postoperative period (72 h)
50–100	Transfuse if:
	Active bleeding
	Neonatal alloimmune thrombocytopenia with intracranial bleed
	Before or after neurosurgical procedure

are not refrigerated, platelets are the blood product most prone to bacterial contamination and have a limited shelf life of 5 days. For the same reason, once a unit of platelets is accessed, it must be transfused within 4 h. They also need to be gently agitated during storage to prevent aggregation [18]. Chilling platelets causes their von Willebrand receptors to cluster and thus activates them. Activated platelets are recognized by macrophages in the liver and are then cleared from plasma rapidly [44]. A dose of 5–10 mL/kg of platelets will raise the plasma platelet count from 50,000/μL to 150,000/μL.

Cryoprecipitate

Cryoprecipitate is prepared by thawing a unit of FFP at 4 °C and removing the plasma to leave the cryoglobulin portion. This cryoglobulin portion is rich in factor VIII (FVIII), factor XIII, fibrinogen, von Willebrand factor (vWF), and fibronectin. The protein is then resuspended in 10–20 mLs of plasma and refrozen within an hour at −18 °C. This smaller volume of cryoprecipitate contains close to the original unit of FFP's amount of fibrinogen, vWF, and factors VIII and XIII – thus allowing rapid replacement of these factors without the additional volume load of FFP.

Indications for cryoprecipitate transfusion are [6, 30]:

1. Hypofibrinogenemia with active bleeding or undergoing an invasive procedure
2. Factor XIII and factor VIII deficiencies with active bleeding or undergoing an invasive procedure in the absence of specific factor concentrates
3. Prior to an invasive procedure, or in bleeding patients with von Willebrand disease (VWD), when desmopressin (DDAVP) is contraindicated or not available and when FVIII concentrate is not available

One unit or 10–20 mLs of cryoprecipitate is sufficient for hemostasis in neonates. A dose of one to two units/10 kg increases plasma fibrinogen levels 60–100 mg/dL. Prior to use, cryoprecipitate is thawed in a water bath at 30–37 °C for 15 min. Thawed cryoprecipitate should be kept at room temperature and used within 6 h after thawing. Once a container of cryoprecipitate is accessed, it should be transfused within 4 h [18].

Fibrinogen Concentrates

In 2009, the Food and Drug Administration (FDA) approved the first fibrinogen concentrate for the treatment of bleeding in patients with congenital fibrinogen deficiency. Fibrinogen concentrate is made from human plasma. The plasma goes through viral inactivation and removal – which inactivates all currently known viruses. Fibrinogen concentrates may thus be safer than nonvirally inactivated cryoprecipitate and FFP. Additionally, fibrinogen concentrate does not need to be screened for blood type and does not need thawing. A large dose can also be administered without an accompanying large volume [45]. Given these benefits, fibrinogen concentrates may be a safe therapeutic option for replacement of fibrinogen, particularly in neonates.

A dose of 70 mg/kg raises fibrinogen levels by 1.0 g/L in the setting of congenital fibrinogen deficiency [46]. There is limited dosing data in the neonatal population. Dosage recommendations are the same as in adults. The dose for fibrinogen concentrates is as follows:

$$\text{Fibrinogen concentrate dose} (g) = \text{Desired increase in plasma fibrinogen level} (g\,/\,L) \\ \times \text{plasma volume} (L)$$

Prothrombin Complex Concentrates

Prothrombin complex concentrates (PCCs) or intermediate purity factor IX concentrates were introduced in the 1970s as a source of factor IX (FIX) for patients with hemophilia B. PCCs contain factors IX, II, and X (three-factor PCCs) and factor VII (four-factor PCCs) – the vitamin K-dependent coagulation factors. They also contain a variable amount of anticoagulant factors, protein C, protein S, and antithrombin. Thrombotic events, such as venous thromboembolism, disseminated intravascular coagulation, and myocardial infarction, have been associated with the use of PCCs in adults, usually when high doses (>200 U/kg/day) were used [47]. PCC use in the treatment of hemophilia B declined after high-purity FIX products were introduced in the 1990s and now with recombinant FIX concentrate. These FIX concentrates are less thrombogenic than PCCs [48]. The administration of PCCs is indicated for prophylaxis and treatment of bleeding in patients with congenital and acquired deficiencies of factors of the prothrombin complex (factors II, VII, IX, and X) in the absence of factor-specific concentrates [49].

As vitamin K-antagonists (VKAs), such as warfarin, have been increasingly used for anticoagulation, so has the need for rapid reversal of VKAs in the setting of major bleeding or emergency surgery. Neonates may also be given VKAs, such as in treatment for homozygous protein C deficiency causing purpura fulminans [50]. In 2013, the FDA approved the first four-factor PCC for the urgent reversal of VKA therapy. For patients taking VKAs with life-threatening bleeds, within 30 min of administration of PCCs, there is sustained replacement of the vitamin K-dependent factors and a decrease in international normalized ratio (INR) to <1.3, when given at an appropriate dose. This effect appears to be more rapid than the reversal that occurs with FFP administration [51]. A dose of 30 mL/kg of FFP is often required to reverse VKAs – introducing a large volume to the patient. Dosing for PCCs is based on international units (IUs) of FIX. One IU of FIX represents the activity of FIX in 1 mL of plasma. In adults, the dosage of PCCs for reversal of a starting INR of 2–6 is 25–50 IU/kg, representing about 1 mL/kg of volume. This may be particularly helpful in neonates, who are at risk for volume overload. PCCs may also be obtained more quickly in an emergency situation, as they do not require blood typing or thawing [51]. It is important to note that the safety and efficacy of PCCs for the reversal of VKAs have not been studied in children or neonates. A recent study has found that PCCs augment thrombin generation in neonatal plasma *ex vivo* after cardiopulmonary bypass [52]. Future studies are needed to evaluate the efficacy and safety of PCCs in neonates.

Antifibrinolytics

Antifibrinolytic agents have been used to minimize blood loss and transfusion, particularly in clinical scenarios with a high likelihood of hyperfibrinolysis. The most notable examples in the neonatal population include cardiac surgery with CPB and neonatal extracorporeal membrane oxygenator (ECMO) support. In both, exposure of blood to a large non-endothelialized artificial surface results in contact activation of the coagulation and fibrinolytic systems. This results in clotting factor consumption, coagulopathy, and exacerbation of ongoing bleeding or spontaneous pathologic bleeding in infants who are already anticoagulated with heparin to prevent thrombosis due to contact with extracorporeal/bypass circuits. Reduced factor concentrations in the neonate and hypothermia during CPB can further worsen hemostatic function.

In the United States, currently available antifibrinolytics include the lysine analogs epsilon-aminocaproic acid (EACA) and tranexamic acid (TXA). The serine protease inhibitor, aprotinin, which has additional anti-inflammatory effects, has also been used in these settings but has been withdrawn from the market due to safety concerns. The lysine analog agents competitively inhibit binding of plasminogen to fibrin, inhibiting formation of the active enzyme plasmin. There is evidence supporting the efficacy of both EACA and TXA for decreasing blood loss and transfusion in pediatric cardiac surgery [53, 54].

The use of antifibrinolytics to prevent hemorrhagic complications in infants and children on ECMO has been explored in a number of studies [55, 56]. The general conclusion of these studies is that antifibrinolytics appear to be safe in this setting and may be useful in reducing bleeding in patients on ECMO undergoing surgical procedures but may not decrease the overall risk of hemorrhagic complications (intracranial hemorrhage).

Vascular Access

The transfusion of blood products in neonates is usually limited to administration via peripheral intravenous catheters (PIV). Peripheral administration of blood via a large bore PIV is preferred in neonates for two major reasons. Firstly, administration of blood through a small-bore catheter may cause hemolysis and associated hyperkalemia. One study in 2004 showed that rapid transfusion of RBCs via a hand-held syringe through 23 gauge or smaller needles caused hemolysis [57]. Secondly, if hyperkalemia or hypocalcemia secondary to citrate toxicity from rapid transfusion occurs, peripheral administration of blood product allows for time for dilution before entering the heart and coronary vessels.

A 22 gauge catheter is considered large bore for a neonate. The antecubital and saphenous veins are among the preferred sites for larger catheter placement [17]. Two randomized, controlled trials have shown that ultrasound-guided PIV placement in pediatric patients with difficult venous access decreases time to successful cannulation [58, 59]. One study showed that ultrasound guidance decreased number of attempts and number of times of needle redirection [59]. This may be particularly beneficial in the preterm neonate with multiple comorbidities, in whom it is important to preserve veins for future peripheral and central venous access.

For prolonged intravenous access, infusion of vasoactive medications, or pressure monitoring, access to the central circulation is preferred. Longer catheters may be placed via the femoral, subclavian, or internal jugular vein. The clinician should carefully choose the length of catheter, taking into consideration that longer catheters produce more resistance to flow and thus are not preferred when relatively rapid infusion of large volumes is required.

Administration Rates

During storage, red blood cells leak potassium into the extracellular fluid. Transfusion-associated hyperkalemic cardiac arrest (TAHCA) has been reported in pediatric patients during massive transfusion or when blood is given at a rate greater than 1.5–2.0 mL/kg/min [17]. Risk factors for TAHCA are massive transfusion of whole blood or PRBCs in a neonate, with blood stored for longer than 7 days, and transfusion via a central venous catheter smaller than 23 gauge [60].

Another complication associated with rapid transfusion is hypocalcemia secondary to citrate toxicity. Citrate, the anticoagulant in stored blood, causes hypocalcemia by binding with ionized calcium (iCa^{2+}). During rapid transfusion, the large load of citrate overwhelms the body's clearance mechanism and begins chelating plasma iCa^{2+}. The rate of infusion of red cells or plasma that produces hypocalcemia is the same as the rate that causes hyperkalemia (1.5–2.0 mL/kg/min). Neonates are at particular risk of citrate toxicity from FFP administration, as FFP has a high plasma and thus citrate load, and a low viscosity, allowing rapid transfusion.

Warmers and Filters

For precise administration of volumes during resuscitation and transfusion of neonates, clinicians may create a stopcock manifold and syringe apparatus. Intravenous tubing is connected to a stopcock manifold. Blood tubing is then connected to the stopcock closest to the patient. A syringe is placed in the stopcock farthest from the patient. The stopcocks are opened to allow blood to fill the syringe and then adjusted to allow accurate volumes to be given from the syringe to the patient. All infusion tubing must be manually de-aired, to prevent iatrogenic venous air embolism, which is a particular concern in infants who may have a persistent patent foramen ovale or persistent ductus arteriosus. In patients with known right-to-left shunts, the use of an in-line air filter is a second safety mechanism that can be used to prevent entrainment of air into the neonate.

Prior to administration, RBCs and FFP need to be warmed in a fluid warmer. A common blood warmer used in neonatal transfusion is the Hotline (Smiths Medical ASD, Rockland, MA), which uses countercurrent heat exchange to rapidly warm fluid along the length of a column of fluid. This can effectively warm blood that is administered up to a rate of 75 mL/min.

All blood component products must be transfused through a filter to remove clots and aggregates prior to administration. A standard 150- to 260-μm filter is used for all blood products. A smaller 20- to 40-μm microaggregate filter may be used when transfusing PRBCs, to remove degenerating platelets, leukocytes, and fibrin strands. However, platelets should only be filtered by large-pore filters (≥150 μm) as micropore filters may adsorb a large number of platelets and thus diminish the effectiveness of platelet transfusion [18].

Perioperative Transfusion Monitoring

Coagulation Monitoring

Perioperative coagulation monitoring is important to diagnose causes of hemorrhage and to guide hemostatic therapies. However, routine coagulation assays such as PT, PTT, international normalized ratio, and fibrinogen do not take into account the contribution of platelets on clot strength and formation. Additionally, these tests may take nearly 60 min to obtain results. Current point-of-care (POC) tests that measure the viscoelastic properties of whole blood include thromboelastography or TEG® (Haemoscope, Niles, IL) and rotation thromboelastometry or ROTEM® (TEM International, Munich, Germany). These tests assess the viscoelastic changes of all phases of clotting whole blood in low sheer settings, including clot formation, thrombin generation, fibrinogen levels, platelet function, and fibrinolysis.

Both TEG® and ROTEM® use similar mechanisms to measure the strength of a blood clot. In TEG®, a thin plastic probe is immersed in a cup with whole blood. The cup moves back and forth in an arc of 4.75° around the plastic pin. As clot begins to form, torque increases between the cup and pin. The change in torque is detected electronically. With ROTEM®, the cup is stationary and the pin rotates back and forth in a 4.75° arc. As clot forms, the change in torque is detected optically. In both techniques, the change in torque is then presented in the form of a tracing.

This section will discuss parameters measured in TEG® assays. ROTEM® has similar parameters, with different nomenclature. TEG® measurements include the time until first evidence of fibrin clot (reaction time, R), the kinetics of fibrin formation and clot development or the time from R until the clot reaches 20 mm (kinetics, k), the slope between R and k (α angle, α), the strength and stability of the fibrin clot (maximum amplitude, MA), and the clot lysis after 30 min ($LY30$) (Fig. 2.1).

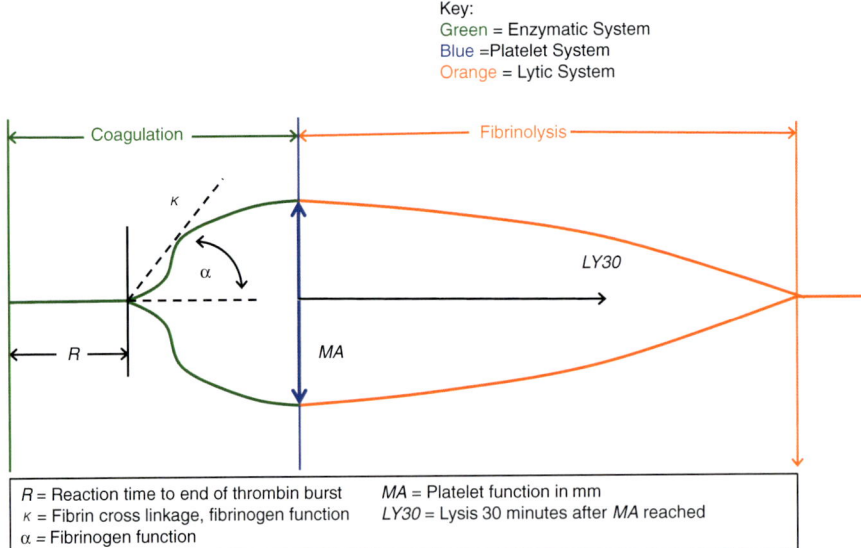

Fig. 2.1 Typical TEG® tracing. R reaction time to end of thrombin burst, k fibrin cross-linkage, fibrinogen function, α fibrinogen function, MA platelet function in mm, $LY30$ lysis 30 min after MA reached

The use of intraoperative thromboelastometry to guide transfusion in pediatric cardiac surgery has been associated with a reduction in proportion of patients receiving transfusions and an altered transfusion pattern. Romlin et al. studied 100 pediatric patients, of an average age of 5–6 months old, and found, in the group of patients where thromboelastometry was used to guide transfusion decisions, significantly fewer patients received PRBCs and FFP, whereas more received platelets and fibrinogen concentrate transfusions [61].

Rapid thromboelastography (r-TEG) is a faster POC assay than TEG®, which can obtain results in 5 min. In r-TEG, tissue factor is added to whole blood, to activate both the intrinsic and extrinsic coagulation pathways.

A generally accepted practice of transfusing blood products in response to the abnormal r-TEG values is as follows [62]:

- With an abnormal ACT or R value, transfuse FFP.
- With an abnormal k time, transfuse cryoprecipitate.
- With an abnormal α angle, transfuse cryoprecipitate.
- With an abnormal MA, transfuse platelets.
- With an elevated $LY30$, administer antifibrinolytics.

Holcomb et al. describe massive transfusion practices at their trauma center of transfusing rapidly bleeding patients in a 1:1:1 ratio of RBCs/FFP/platelets. Once bleeding has slowed, they transition to thromboelastography-guided transfusion therapy to replace specific blood components [63].

Summary

Neonates have special physiologic and pathophysiologic considerations in relation to blood component transfusion. Preterm neonates, in particular, are at high risk of requiring transfusions in their first weeks of life. Clinicians involved in the care of neonates need a thorough understanding of blood components and indications for transfusion in this patient population. For each patient and clinical scenario, the provider must use their clinical judgment in deciding need for transfusion and the appropriate product, access, and monitoring required.

References

1. Fabres J, Wehrli G, Marques MB, Phillips V, Dimmitt RA, Westfall AO, et al. Estimating blood needs for very-low-birth-weight infants. Transfusion. 2006;46(11):1915–20.
2. Christensen RD, Carroll PD, Josephson CD. Evidence-based advances in transfusion practice in neonatal intensive care units. Neonatology. 2014;106(3):245–53.
3. Oh W, Fanaroff AA, Carlo WA, Donovan EF, McDonald SA, Poole WK. Effects of delayed cord clamping in very-low-birth-weight infants. J Perinatol. 2011;31:S68–71.
4. Rabe H, Diaz-Rossello JL, Duley L, Dowswell T. Effect of timing of umbilical cord clamping and other strategies to influence placental transfusion at preterm birth on maternal and infant

outcomes. Rabe H, editor. Cochrane Database Syst Rev. Chichester: John Wiley & Sons, Ltd; 2012;8:CD003248.

5. Josephson CD, Glynn SA, Kleinman SH, Blajchman MA. A multidisciplinary "think tank": the top 10 clinical trial opportunities in transfusion medicine from the National Heart, Lung, and Blood Institute-sponsored 2009 state-of-the-science symposium. Transfusion. 2010;51(4):828–41.

6. Roseff SD, Luban NLC, Manno CS. Guidelines for assessing appropriateness of pediatric transfusion. Transfusion. 2002;42(11):1398–413.

7. Kelly AM, Williamson LM. Neonatal transfusion. Early Hum Dev. 2013;89(11):855–60.

8. Venkatesh V, Khan R, Curley A, New H, Stanworth S. How we decide when a neonate needs a transfusion. Br J Haematol. 2012;160(4):421–33.

9. Bednarek FJ, Weisberger S, Richardson DK, Frantz ID, Shah B, Rubin LP. Variations in blood transfusions among newborn intensive care units. SNAP II Study Group. J Pediatr. 1998;133(5):601–7.

10. Guillén U, Cummings JJ, Bell EF, Hosono S, Frantz AR, Maier RF, et al. International survey of transfusion practices for extremely premature infants. Semin Perinatol. 2012;36(4):244–7.

11. Lacroix J, Hébert PC, Hutchison JS, Hume HA, Tucci M, Ducruet T, et al. Transfusion strategies for patients in pediatric intensive care units. N Engl J Med. 2007;356(16):1609–19.

12. Lacroix J, Demaret P, Tucci M. Red blood cell transfusion: decision making in pediatric intensive care units. Semin Perinatol. 2012;36(4):225–31.

13. Hébert PC, Wells G, Blajchman MA, Marshall J, Martin C, Pagliarello G, et al. A multicenter, randomized, controlled clinical trial of transfusion requirements in critical care. Transfusion Requirements in Critical Care Investigators, Canadian Critical Care Trials Group. N Engl J Med. 1999;340(6):409–17.

14. Bell EF, Strauss RG, Widness JA, Mahoney LT, Mock DM, Seward VJ, et al. Randomized trial of liberal versus restrictive guidelines for red blood cell transfusion in preterm infants. Pediatrics. 2005;115(6):1685–91.

15. Kirpalani H, Whyte RK, Andersen C, Asztalos EV, Heddle N, Blajchman MA, et al. The premature infants in need of transfusion (pint) study: a randomized, controlled trial of a restrictive (low) versus liberal (high) transfusion threshold for extremely low birth weight infants. J Pediatr. 2006;149(3):301–3.

16. Whyte R, Kirpalani H. Low versus high haemoglobin concentration threshold for blood transfusion for preventing morbidity and mortality in very low birth weight infants. Cochrane Database Syst Rev. 2011;(11):CD000512.

17. Cote CJ, Lerman J, Anderson BJ. A practice of anesthesia for infants and children. 5th ed. Philadelphia: Elsevier Health Sciences; 2013.

18. Roback JD, Mark K, Fung E, Grossman BJ, Hillyer CD. Technical manual. 18th ed. Bethesda: American Association of Blood Banks; 2014.

19. Repine TB, Perkins JG, Kauvar DS, Blackborne L. The use of fresh whole blood in massive transfusion. J Trauma Injury Infect Crit Care. 2006;60(Supplement):S59–69.

20. Spinella PC. Warm fresh whole blood transfusion for severe hemorrhage: U.S. military and potential civilian applications. Crit Care Med. 2008;36(7 Suppl):S340–5.

21. Miller RD, Robbins TO, Tong MJ, Barton SL. Coagulation defects associated with massive blood transfusions. Ann Surg. 1971;174(5):794–801.

22. Spinella PC, Perkins JG, Grathwohl KW, Beekley AC, Holcomb JB. Warm fresh whole blood is independently associated with improved survival for patients with combat-related traumatic injuries. J Trauma. 2009;66(4 Suppl):S69–76.

23. Kiraly LN, Underwood S, Differding JA, Schreiber MA. Transfusion of aged packed red blood cells results in decreased tissue oxygenation in critically injured trauma patients. J Trauma Injury Infect Crit Care. 2009;67(1):29–32.

24. Jobes DR, Sesok-Pizzini D, Friedman D. Reduced transfusion requirement with use of fresh whole blood in pediatric cardiac surgical procedures. Ann Thorac Surg. 2015;99(5):1706–11.

25. Mou SS, Giroir BP, Molitor-Kirsch EA, Leonard SR, Nikaidoh H, Nizzi F, et al. Fresh whole blood versus reconstituted blood for pump priming in heart surgery in infants. N Engl J Med. 2004;351(16):1635–44.
26. Gruenwald CE, McCrindle BW, Crawford-Lean L, Holtby H, Parshuram C, Massicotte P, et al. Reconstituted fresh whole blood improves clinical outcomes compared with stored component blood therapy for neonates undergoing cardiopulmonary bypass for cardiac surgery: a random-ized controlled trial. J Thorac Cardiovasc Surg. 2008;136(6):1442–9.
27. Stricker PA, Fiadjoe JE, Davis AR, Sussman E, Burgess BJ, Ciampa B, et al. Reconstituted blood reduces blood donor exposures in children undergoing craniofacial reconstruction sur-gery. Paediatr Anaesth. 2011;21(1):54–61.
28. Ness PM, Pennington RM. Plasma fractionation in the United States: a review for clinicians. JAMA. 1974;230(2):247.
29. Motta M, Vecchio AD, Chirico G. Fresh frozen plasma administration in the neonatal intensive care unit. Clin Perinatol. 2015;42(3):639–50.
30. British Committee for Standards in Haematology, Blood Transfusion Task Force Duguid J, O'Shaughnessy DF, Atterbury C, Bolton Maggs P, Murphy M, Thomas D, et al. Guidelines for the use of fresh-frozen plasma, cryoprecipitate and cryosupernatant. Br J Haematol. 2004;126(1):11–28.
31. Girelli G, Antoncecchi S, Casadei AM, Del Vecchio A, Isernia P, Motta M, et al. Recommendations for transfusion therapy in neonatology. Blood Transfus. 2015;13(3):484–97.
32. Randomised trial of prophylactic early fresh-frozen plasma or gelatin or glucose in preterm babies: outcome at 2 years. Lancet. 1996;348(9022):229–32.
33. Christensen RD, Baer VL, Lambert DK, Henry E, Ilstrup SJ, Bennett ST. Reference intervals for common coagulation tests of preterm infants (CME). Transfusion. 2013;54(3):627–32.
34. Yazer MH, Cortese-Hassett A, Triulzi DJ. Coagulation factor levels in plasma frozen within 24 hours of phlebotomy over 5 days of storage at 1 to 6°C. Transfusion. 2008;48(12):2525–30.
35. von Heymann C, Keller MK, Spies C, Schuster M, Meinck K, Sander M, et al. Activity of clot-ting factors in fresh-frozen plasma during storage at 4 degrees C over 6 days. Transfusion. 2009;49(5):913–20.
36. Del Vecchio A, Motta M. Evidence-based platelet transfusion recommendations in neonates. J Matern Fetal Neonatal Med. 2011;24 Suppl 1:38–40.
37. Josephson CD, Su LL, Christensen RD, Hillyer CD, Castillejo M-I, Emory MR, et al. Platelet transfusion practices among neonatologists in the United States and Canada: results of a sur-vey. Pediatrics. 2009;123(1):278–85.
38. Cremer M, Sola-Visner M, Roll S, Josephson CD, Yilmaz Z, Bührer C, et al. Platelet transfu-sions in neonates: practices in the United States vary significantly from those in Austria, Germany, and Switzerland. Transfusion. 2011;51(12):2634–41.
39. Christensen RD, Henry E, Wiedmeier SE, Stoddard RA, Sola-Visner MC, Lambert DK, et al. Thrombocytopenia among extremely low birth weight neonates: data from a multihospital healthcare system. J Perinatol. 2006;26(6):348–53.
40. Andrew M, Castle V, Saigal S, Carter C, Kelton JG. Clinical impact of neonatal thrombocyto-penia. J Pediatr. 1987;110(3):457–64.
41. Muthukumar P, Venkatesh V, Curley A, Kahan BC, Choo L, Ballard S, et al. Severe thrombo-cytopenia and patterns of bleeding in neonates: results from a prospective observational study and implications for use of platelet transfusions. Transfus Med. 2012;22(5):338–43.
42. Andrew M, Vegh P, Caco C, Kirpalani H, Jefferies A, Ohlsson A, et al. A randomized, con-trolled trial of platelet transfusions in thrombocytopenic premature infants. J Pediatr. 1993;123(2):285–91.
43. Sparger K, Deschmann E, Sola-Visner M. Platelet transfusions in the neonatal intensive care unit. Clin Perinatol. 2015;42(3):613–23.
44. Hoffmeister KM, Felbinger TW, Falet H, Denis CV, Bergmeier W, Mayadas TN, et al. The clearance mechanism of chilled blood platelets. Cell. 2003;112(1):87–97.

45. Levy JH, Welsby I, Goodnough LT. Fibrinogen as a therapeutic target for bleeding: a review of critical levels and replacement therapy. Transfusion. 2014;54(5):1389–405.
46. Kreuz W, Meili E, Peter-Salonen K, Haertel S, Devay J, Krzensk U, et al. Efficacy and tolerability of a pasteurised human fibrinogen concentrate in patients with congenital fibrinogen deficiency. Transfus Apher Sci. 2005;32(3):247–53.
47. Dusel CH, Grundmann C, Eich S, Seitz R, Konig H. Identification of prothrombin as a major thrombogenic agent in prothrombin complex concentrates. Blood Coagul Fibrinolysis. 2004;15(5):405–11.
48. Key NS, Negrier C. Coagulation factor concentrates: past, present, and future. Lancet. 2007;370(9585):439–48.
49. Williams MD, Chalmers EA, Gibson BES, Haemostasis and Thrombosis Task Force, British Committee for Standards in Haematology. The investigation and management of neonatal haemostasis and thrombosis. Br J Haematol. 2002;119:295–309.
50. Monagle P, Chan AKC, Goldenberg NA, Ichord RN, Journeycake JM, Nowak-Göttl U, et al. Antithrombotic therapy in neonates and children: antithrombotic therapy and prevention of thrombosis, 9th ed: American College of Chest Physicians evidence-based clinical practice guidelines. Chest. 2012;141(2 Suppl):e737S–801S.
51. Colomina MJ, Díez Lobo A, Garutti I, Gómez-Luque A, Llau JV, Pita E. Perioperative use of prothrombin complex concentrates. Minerva Anestesiol. 2012;78(3):358–68.
52. Guzzetta NA, Szlam F, Kiser AS, Fernandez JD, Szlam AD, Leong T, et al. Augmentation of thrombin generation in neonates undergoing cardiopulmonary bypass. Br J Anaesth. 2014;112(2):319–27.
53. Lin C-Y, Shuhaiber JH, Loyola H, Liu H, del Nido P, DiNardo JA, et al. The safety and efficacy of antifibrinolytic therapy in neonatal cardiac surgery. PLoS One. 2015;10(5), e0126514.
54. Eaton MP. Antifibrinolytic therapy in surgery for congenital heart disease. Anesth Analg. 2008;106(4):1087–100.
55. Horwitz JR, Cofer BR, Warner BW, Cheu HW, Lally KP. A multicenter trial of 6-aminocaproic acid (Amicar) in the prevention of bleeding in infants on ECMO. J Pediatr Surg. 1998;33(11):1610–3.
56. Downard CD, Betit P, Chang RW, Garza JJ, Arnold JH, Wilson JM. Impact of Amicar on hemorrhagic complications of ECMO: a ten-year review. J Pediatr Surg. 2003;38(8):1212–6.
57. Miller MA, Schlueter AJ. Transfusions via hand-held syringes and small-gauge needles as risk factors for hyperkalemia. Transfusion. 2004;44(3):373–81.
58. Benkhadra M, Collignon M, Fournel I, Oeuvrard C, Rollin P, Perrin M, et al. Ultrasound guidance allows faster peripheral IV cannulation in children under 3 years of age with difficult venous access: a prospective randomized study. Paediatr Anaesth. 2012;22(5):449–54.
59. Doniger SJ, Ishimine P, Fox JC, Kanegaye JT. Randomized controlled trial of ultrasound-guided peripheral intravenous catheter placement versus traditional techniques in difficult-access pediatric patients. Pediatr Emerg Care. 2009;25(3):154–9.
60. Lee AC, Reduque LL, Luban NLC, Ness PM, Anton B, Heitmiller ES. Transfusion-associated hyperkalemic cardiac arrest in pediatric patients receiving massive transfusion. Transfusion. 2013;54(1):244–54.
61. Romlin BS, Wåhlander H, Berggren H, Synnergren M, Baghaei F, Nilsson K, et al. Intraoperative thromboelastometry is associated with reduced transfusion prevalence in pediatric cardiac surgery. Anesth Analg. 2011;112(1):30–6.
62. Kashuk JL, Moore EE, Le T, Lawrence J, Pezold M, Johnson JL, et al. Noncitrated whole blood is optimal for evaluation of postinjury coagulopathy with point-of-care rapid thrombelastography. J Surg Res. 2009;156(1):133–8.
63. Holcomb JB, Minei KM, Scerbo ML, Radwan ZA, Wade CE, Kozar RA, et al. Admission rapid thrombelastography can replace conventional coagulation tests in the emergency department. Ann Surg. 2012;256(3):476–86.

Chapter 3
Special Disease Considerations in the Neonate

Michele P. Lambert

Introduction

Neonates, because of their unique status of transitioning from fetal to independent living, deserve special consideration with regard to transfusion for typical blood and coagulation parameters. Most adult laboratory values are fairly stable over time; in contrast, neonatal reference ranges change significantly over the first few days of life and vary with gestational age and birth weight. These values, especially for coagulation factors, may not reach normal adult levels, for 6–12 months. In this chapter, we will discuss the major hematologic abnormalities encountered in the newborn that may require transfusion intervention and a basic approach to their evaluation/management. However, as each of these concepts could easily be a chapter unto themselves, the discussion will be in fairly broad strokes, and the reader will be referred to other sources for further reading.

M.P. Lambert, MD, MTR
The Children's Hospital of Philadelphia, Division of Hematology, Department of Pediatrics, Philadelphia, PA, USA

Perelman School of Medicine University of Pennsylvania, Department of Pediatrics, Philadelphia, PA, USA
e-mail: lambertm@email.chop.edu

© Springer International Publishing Switzerland 2017   47
D.A. Sesok-Pizzini (ed.), *Neonatal Transfusion Practices*,
DOI 10.1007/978-3-319-42764-5_3

Anemia

Definition of Anemia

The hemoglobin value at which a neonate is deemed anemic depends on both gestational age and birth weight [1]. Generally, anemia is defined as hemoglobin or hematocrit >2 SD below the mean for postnatal age [2] and is a common problem in newborns in the neonatal intensive care unit (NICU). In fact almost 50% of neonates in the NICU require transfusion, and 90% of extremely low-birth-weight infants (infants weighing <1000 g) require at least one transfusion of red blood cells (RBC) [3]. In addition, there are several variables, beyond the gestational age, that may influence the hemoglobin at the time of delivery which include conduct of labor, treatment of the umbilical vessels, and site and time of blood sampling (cord blood, capillary, or venous samples) [2].

A basic approach to the anemic neonate and several reference guidelines for transfusion management are presented. Transfusion practice guidelines have been proposed for management of preterm neonates [4] (and have changed over recent years as our understanding of the important changes in the preterm neonate has increased), although several controversies still exist about optimal management of these small and often critically ill neonates [3, 5]. In contrast, the management of well term neonates has been relatively stable [2].

Approach to the Anemic Neonate

In considering the anemic neonate, it is useful to think about the ways in which a neonate may become anemic. In general, these are not different from the ways in which any patient may become anemic (Table 3.1): blood loss, decreased production, or red cell destruction. Therefore, the approach to anemic neonate is similar to any other anemic patient, but the patient's personal medical history is significantly shorter and family history and maternal medical history play a much more important role in aiding in the diagnosis.

In obtaining a family history, it is important to ask about a history of jaundice, gallstones, transfusions, splenomegaly or splenectomy, and iron supplementation. The maternal obstetric history should include fetal growth, viral infections, placental or cord pathology, fetal distress, and method of delivery. Physical exam should not only assess for evidence of pallor or jaundice but also for hepatosplenomegaly, tachycardia, and associated congenital malformations that may provide a clue to congenital anemias. Diagnostic laboratory evaluation should include complete blood count (CBC), reticulocyte and nucleated red blood cell counts, evaluation of the red blood cell indices and the peripheral smear as well as serum bilirubin and lactate dehydrogenase levels (to look for evidence of hemolysis), and a direct antiglobulin test (Coombs test) to measure the presence of antibodies directed against red blood cells. The laboratory evaluation in combination with physical exam and history can guide the clinician to the correct diagnosis, and the clinical evaluation with the hemoglobin can help guide transfusion.

Table 3.1 Causes of anemia in the newborn period

Blood loss	
Occult blood loss prior to delivery	Fetomaternal hemorrhage
	Twin to twin transfusion
Obstetric causes	Abruptio placentae
	Placenta previa
	Rupture cord
	Cesarean section
	Intrauterine manipulation
	Incision of placenta at C-section
Internal hemorrhage in neonate	Intracranial
	Retroperitoneal
	Ruptured spleen or liver
	Giant cephalohematoma
	GI bleeding
Increased destruction (hemolysis)	
Hereditary RBC disorders	RBC membrane disorders (spherocytosis, elliptocytosis, etc.)
	Enzymopathies (G6PD deficiency, PK deficiency)
	Hemoglobinopathies (α or γ thalassemias)
Immune	ABO incompatibility
	Rh incompatibility
	Minor blood group incompatibility
	Maternal autoimmune disease (AIHA, lupus)
	Drug induced
Acquired	Infection
	DIC
	Microangiopathic hemolytic anemia (renal artery stenosis, cavernous hemangioma)
	Nutritional (vitamin E)
Decreased production	
	Physiologic anemia of infancy
	Anemia of prematurity
	Diamond-Blackfan anemia
	Trisomy 21
	Pearson syndrome
	Osteopetrosis
	Drug induced
	Infection (parvovirus B19, CMV, adenovirus)

Guidelines for Transfusion Practice

Generally, transfusions should be considered for infants who are symptomatic from anemia. The most common transfusions given in neonates are given to premature infants who are either in the very low-birth-weight (VLBW) or extremely low-birth-weight (ELBW) categories as these two groups of infants are at increased risk for

Table 3.2 Transfusion guidelines for VLBW infants based on hemoglobin level (g/dL)

Age (days)	Sample type	Receiving respiratory support	Not receiving respiratory support
1–7	Capillary	≤11.5	≤10
	Venous	≤10.4	≤9
8–14	Capillary	≤10	≤8.5
	Venous	≤9	≤7.7
≥15	Capillary	≤8.5	≤7.5
	Venous	≤7.7	≤6.8

anemia of prematurity. Generally, efforts are directed at limiting phlebotomy in preterm infants and at maximizing initial blood volume with delayed cord clamping [4]. Efforts to decrease early transfusions (during the first postnatal days) and reduce donor exposures and number of total transfusions have led to fairly restrictive transfusion practices in the NICU, partly due to concerns about risks of grade 3 or 4 intraventricular hemorrhage [6] and necrotizing enterocolitis (NEC) [7]. However, concern remains about long-term neurodevelopmental outcomes in withholding transfusion, and so ongoing prospective clinical trials are warranted to address optimal transfusion practices [8]. Current guidelines (Tables 3.2 and 3.3) recommend transfusion thresholds based on postnatal age, birth weight, and need for respiratory support in infants who are not exhibiting hemodynamic evidence of anemia (tachycardia/tachypnea/shock) [10]. In the setting of severe neonatal anemia (hemoglobin ≤8 g/dL at birth) or associated with hypovolemic shock (generally associated with a ≥20 % volume loss) due to bleeding, the neonate should be transfused with red cells to correct the anticipated volume loss. In the setting of symptomatic anemia that develops after birth where the hemoglobin is below reference values for age and the infant has symptoms of anemia, transfusion should be performed to alleviate symptomatic anemia.

Generally, simple transfusion is the best choice of transfusion for most neonates with anemia. Occasionally, an exchange transfusion may be indicated as in the setting of hemolytic disease of the newborn where the bilirubin is very high (within 9–12 h of birth >5 mg/dL) or the cord blood hemoglobin is low (≤8 g/dL) or in rare cases of severe anemia and hyperbilirubinemia associated with sepsis, prematurity, glucose-6-phosphate deficiency, acidosis, or hypoalbuminemia [10]. In contrast, partial exchange transfusion may be indicated in settings of congestive heart failure associated with more chronic anemia as seen in hemolytic disease of the newborn with hydrops or in chronic fetal-maternal hemorrhage or in twin-to-twin transfusion syndrome as this allows for the correction of hemoglobin without substantial changes in blood volume [10].

In conclusion, the causes of neonatal anemia are quite varied, and the management of neonatal anemia varies and may include careful observation and minimizing phlebotomy to transfusion. Careful assessment of the infant and determination of the underlying cause of the anemia is crucial in helping to guide the management. Hemolytic disease of the newborn was not covered in this chapter as it is dealt with elsewhere in this volume.

Table 3.3 Transfusion guidelines for patients aged <4 months [9]

Hct <20% with *low reticulocyte count* and symptoms of anemia[a]
Hct <30% with an infant:
On <35% oxygen by hood
On continuous positive airway pressure and/or intermittent mandatory ventilation with mechanical ventilation with mean airway pressure <6 cm H_2O
With significant apnea or bradycardia[b]
With significant tachycardia or tachypnea[c]
With poor weight gain[d]
Hct <35% with an infant:
On >35% oxygen by hood
On continuous positive airway pressure/intermittent mandatory ventilation with mean airway pressure ≥6–8 cm H_2O
Hct <45% with an infant:
On ECMO
With congenital cyanotic heart disease

[a]Tachycardia, tachypnea, poor feeding
[b]More than six episodes in 12 h or two episodes in 24 h requiring bag and mask ventilation while on methylxanthines
[c]Heart rate >180 beats/min for 24 h, respiratory rate >80 breaths per min for 24 h
[d]Gain of <10 g/day observed over 4 days while receiving ≥100 kcal/kg/day

Polycythemia

Definition of Polycythemia

In contrast to the anemic neonate, polycythemia represents an overabundance of hemoglobin and is defined as a venous hematocrit ≥65% (in a term neonate) or >2 SD above the normal value for gestational age. This is a fairly rare occurrence in infants and is observed in 0.4–4% of neonates [11].

Approach to the Polycythemic Neonate

Generally, polycythemia can be caused by either active erythropoiesis (i.e., transient myeloproliferative disorder associated with trisomy 21, placental insufficiency, maternal diabetes) or passive transfusion (i.e., delayed cord clamping and twin-twin transfusion syndrome). Infants with chronic hypoxia have a higher incidence and premature infants (<34 weeks gestation) rarely have polycythemia [12]. Concern regarding polycythemia stems from hyperviscosity and the attendant risk for micro-circulatory complications including cerebral ischemia and end-organ damage. Predicting which children will have complications, however, is challenging as clinical signs of hyperviscosity are non-specific and may be associated with other clinical contexts but include jitteriness, lethargy, hypotonia, respiratory distress, hypoglycemia, and cyanosis. Additionally, polycythemia is associated with conditions that cause chronic intrauterine hypoxia (maternal diabetes, smoking, hyperthyroidism, hypertension, preeclampsia, placental insufficiency, and intrauterine growth restriction) [13], so how much of the long-term sequelae are due to polycythemia and how much due to intrauterine changes is difficult to parse out [14]. The increase in red cell mass also results in increased bilirubin load to the immature liver resulting in an elevated risk of hyperbilirubinemia in approximately one third of infants [15].

Guidelines for Transfusion Practice

Treatment for polycythemia is controversial. Previous recommendations suggested partial volume exchange transfusion for symptomatic infants with polycythemia (suggesting hyperviscosity) and hematocrit >65 % and even for many asymptomatic infants with hematocrit >70 % [12]. However, recently, some sources have suggested more restrictive management with hydration and supportive care [16] as the first line of therapy for polycythemic infants with partial exchange transfusion as an alternative treatment because of the equivocal data on benefits of partial exchange transfusion for management [17].

Thrombocytopenia

Definition of Thrombocytopenia

Thrombocytopenia is a common problem in the NICU but not typical in healthy term neonates. Thrombocytopenia occurs in <1 % of healthy neonates [18] but 18–35 % of infants in the intensive care unit [19]. It is defined as a platelet count $<150 \times 10^9/L$. Preterm infants may have, as a matter of course, lower platelet counts than term infants, but establishing "normal" platelet counts is difficult in this population because so many of these infants have underlying other illness. The majority of infants with thrombocytopenia are asymptomatic and do not have significant bleeding, and the degree of thrombocytopenia postnatally may not predict risk. However, sometimes profound bleeding, even devastating intracranial hemorrhage (ICH), may result in significant morbidity and mortality.

Approach to the Thrombocytopenic Neonate

Similar to anemia, the causes of thrombocytopenia can be broadly classified into three main categories: increased destruction, increased consumption (loss), or decreased production. For thrombocytopenia, it is useful also to consider the timing

Early onset			Late onset	
Maternal causes	Well baby	Sick baby	Relatively well baby	Sick baby
• Preeclampsia/pregnancy induced HTN • IUGR • Placental insufficiency • Diabetes • HELLP	• Sepsis • FNAIT • Aotoimmune (ITP/Lupus) • Alloimmune hepatitis	• Sepsis • TORCH • DIC • Asphyxia • Chromosomal anomaly	• Thrombosis (renal vein, catheter related) • Medication	• Infection (bacterial/fungal) • NEC
	• hemolytic disease related			
• Consider rare causes for prolonged duration (>7–10 days) such as inherited thrombocytopenia, bone marrow failure syndromes, pulmonary hypertension			• Consider rare causes for prolonged duration (>7–10 days) such as inherited thrombocytopenia, bone marrow failure syndromes, pulmonary hypertension	

Fig. 3.1 Approach to the thrombocytopenic neonate based on onset of low platelet count

of onset of the thrombocytopenia as this helps to differentiate, to some degree, the potential causes: early-onset (within 72 h of birth) versus late-onset thrombocytopenia (occurring after the first 72 h after birth) (Fig. 3.1).

Fetal/Neonatal Alloimmune Thrombocytopenia In thrombocytopenic neonates who are otherwise well and fairly asymptomatic, except for perhaps some petechiae, with early-onset, severe thrombocytopenia, the most likely etiology is increased destruction caused by fetal/neonatal alloimmune thrombocytopenia (FNAIT). This occurs in 1 in 1000–1 in 5000 live births [20] and may cause profound thrombocytopenia with 90 % of infants having platelet counts $<50 \times 10^9$/L and 50 % of infants with platelet counts $<20 \times 10^9$/L [20] suggested by some authors. However, a population screening study in Norway suggests that more mild forms of this disorder also exist and may be easily overlooked, particularly in relatively asymptomatic infants with platelet counts $>50 \times 10^9$/L [21]. This thrombocytopenia is generally fairly short-lived postnatally and resolves fairly quickly after delivery, generally within 1–2 weeks. ICH occurs in up to 20 % of FNAIT [22] making it the most common cause of ICH in term newborns [20]. Some patients are at increased risk for ICH, but to date, the best predictor of a subsequent pregnancy with a fetus with intracranial hemorrhage is a previous pregnancy with ICH [23]. Unlike hemolytic disease of the newborn, FNAIT may occur with the first pregnancy [24] and tends to be more severe with subsequent pregnancies [25]. The severity of FNAIT is also associated with maternal HLA type such that women who are HPA-1a negative and have the HLA DRB3*0101+ allele are 140 times more likely to develop antibodies than women with the HLA DRB3*0101- allele [26].

While some infants with FNAIT have few initial symptoms, many exhibit significant bleeding after delivery. ICH may lead to neurological impairment and significant morbidity and is associated with up to 5 % mortality [22]. Therefore, neonates with suspected FNAIT often receive platelet transfusions to rapidly increase the platelet count. Since FNAIT is due to maternal antibodies directed against fetal platelet antigens that are inherited from the father and lacking the mother [27], the ideal platelet transfusion is with donor-matched, antigen-negative platelets [28], and HPA-1a- and HPA-5b-negative platelets will be compatible in up to 95 % of neonates with FNAIT [29]. However, platelet transfusion should not be delayed to obtain matched platelets, since unmatched platelets can be just as effective [30]. Alternatively, treatment with IVIG has also been used and may offer some benefit when platelet transfusion is not available [22] and may reduce the number of transfusions needed [31, 32].

Other Thrombocytopenias In contrast, the thrombocytopenia due to maternal immune thrombocytopenia (ITP) is generally less severe, and 8–13 % of infants show platelet counts $<50 \times 10^9/L$ [33]. Intracranial hemorrhage is less common in this setting, occurring in only 0–2.9 % of neonates [34], reflecting a possible difference in pathophysiology. Risk factors for severe thrombocytopenia, however, again include a sibling with severe thrombocytopenia [35, 36] and a maternal history of refractory ITP (defined as requiring splenectomy for management) [34, 35, 37]. Additionally, while infants born with FNAIT generally have their lowest platelet count at birth or shortly after birth (within 24–48 h), infants of mothers with ITP continue to drop their platelet counts for 2–4 days after delivery and may remain thrombocytopenic for significantly longer, sometimes even a few months as with hemolytic disease of the newborn [24]. Treatment with IVIG may be sufficient in these infants unless thrombocytopenia is severe [38].

Other causes of early-onset thrombocytopenia may be due to decreased production of platelets by the neonate such as those thrombocytopenias that are associated with maternal causes: placental insufficiency, intrauterine growth retardation, eclampsia, HELLP syndrome, and maternal diabetes [19]. Additionally, various fetal infections such as the "TORCH" infections (*Toxoplasma gondii*, rubella, herpes simplex, HIV, and CMV) can cause severe, early-onset thrombocytopenia. At least one third of CMV infected and 20 % of infants infected with toxoplasma will have severe thrombocytopenia [39]. Finally, severe infection (sepsis) needs to be excluded, as do rare causes such as the inherited thrombocytopenias and certain aneuploidies [12].

In contrast, late-onset, precipitous drop in platelet count is associated with high risk of bleeding and should prompt immediate evaluation for sepsis (bacterial or fungal), necrotizing enterocolitis (NEC), drug-induced thrombocytopenia, and thrombosis (particularly if a central venous or arterial catheter is in place) [19]. The first two etiologies are more common.

Guidelines for Transfusion Practice

A prospective observational trial showed that the 18 % of premature (<34 week gestation) neonates with severe thrombocytopenia (defined as a platelet count $<60 \times 10^9/L$) died or had major bleeding during the study [40], but there was no clear relationship between platelet count and bleeding, and 91 % of infants with platelet count $<20 \times 10^9$/L had no bleeding. Transfusion thresholds in neonates have never been assessed in randomized clinical trials (although an ongoing randomized clinical trial is recruiting in the UK [41]). Because of this, transfusion guidelines vary widely with clinical practice [42]. However, several studies have failed to demonstrate increased risk of intraventricular hemorrhage when platelet transfusion thresholds were restrictive in the setting of severe thrombocytopenia in neonates [43, 44]. In general, the USA and Canada use more liberal transfusion thresholds [45], often transfusing infants with platelet counts $\geq 50 \times 10^9$/L, while the UK tended to use a more restrictive threshold of 25×10^9/L in term and 30×10^9/L in preterm neonates [40].

Neutropenia

Definition of Neutropenia

The absolute neutrophil count (ANC) can be calculated by multiplying the % neutrophils (+ any reported % bands) x WBC count. Neutropenia is seen in about 8 % of NICU admissions [46, 47]. Statistically, neutropenia is defined as a neutrophil count <2 SD below the mean value for gestational age and postnatal age [48]. Practically, however, neutropenia is probably most relevant with neutrophil counts <1000/mcL, although the relationship between low ANC and the risk of infection has not been well established. An absolute neutrophil count of <500/mcL may be more associated with increased risk of infection, especially when persisting for multiple days [49, 50]. In VLBW infants, the risk of infection and the mortality attributable to neutropenic infection is higher than in term neonates [51].

Approach to the Neutropenic Neonate

The same basic mechanisms of neutropenia exist as for the other cytopenias: decreased production, increased destruction, or increased consumption (loss). In critically ill and premature neonates, the causes of neonatal neutropenia are similar to those of neonatal thrombocytopenia: maternal hypertension (decreased production) [52], neonatal sepsis and twin-twin transfusion syndrome (most likely consumption/loss) [53], alloimmunization [54], and hemolytic disease (most likely destruction) [48]. Typically, neutropenia is self-limited and resolves with the underlying cause in these infants [51], but occasionally, it can be prolonged and predispose to serious bacterial infection or may be the clue to significant underlying diseases such as bone marrow failure syndromes and requires careful investigation [55].

The most common cause of neutropenia lasting >24 h in neonates is maternal pregnancy-induced hypertension where neutropenia occurs in 49 % of infants [52].

The mechanism may be decreased neutrophil production in this setting and correlates with degree of growth restriction and placental insufficiency. This correlation has been shown in several studies which also noted that VLBW and small for gestational age infants may be at increased risk for more severe neutropenia, although the role of this neutropenia and its role in infant mortality and sepsis are still not clear [24].

Neonatal Alloimmune Neutropenia (NAN) NAN occurs in 0.2–2% of neonates, although the true incidence is not known because not all infants have a CBC and this entity may be asymptomatic [56]. Alloimmune neutropenia, like alloimmune thrombocytopenia, occurs because of maternal sensitization to paternal antigens on neonatal neutrophils. Fetomaternal incompatibility occurs in about 20% of pregnancies [57], however, and alloimmunization occurs in 0.6–1.1% of pregnancies [57, 58]. Like FNAIT, this is a transient phenomenon but lasts between 1 and 4 months [59]. Data on the incidence of infection is limited as there are very few prospective studies. A recent study from the Netherlands examined 35 cases of NAN and found that more than half of the infants presented with infection (21/35), but all of them responded to treatment with antibiotics only [56]. Other studies suggest an incidence of infections of 20% (1 out of 5) [54].

The association of neutropenia with other cytopenias (thrombocytopenia, anemia) may indicate several etiologies (hemolytic disease, maternal hypertension, maternal diabetes, or sepsis) but may also be a sign of bone marrow failure and should be carefully monitored. Prolonged multilineage cytopenias (>2 weeks) should prompt consideration of a bone marrow biopsy because only 10% of neutropenic babies will remain so for this long [52], as should profound neutropenia or neutropenia that fails to respond to treatment with G-CSF as immune thrombocytopenia generally corrects with G-CSF [60].

Guidelines for Transfusion Practice

Unlike other cytopenias, neutropenia cannot easily be managed with transfusion as granulocyte infusions carry significant risks not present in transfusion of other products and are not easily available. They are generally considered experimental or a treatment of last resort. A Cochrane analysis concluded that further studies are warranted to determine whether granulocyte infusions are useful in the setting of severe neonatal sepsis with neutropenia [61]. Any neonate with neutropenia should be immediately evaluated for sepsis as this is the most likely etiology, particularly in an ill neonate. Recombinant granulocyte colony-stimulating factor (G-CSF) and granulocyte-macrophage colony-stimulating factor (GM-CSF) may be used to treat neonatal neutropenia. G-CSF stimulates neutrophil production and release from the bone marrow, while GM-CSF can stimulate both neutrophil and macrophage production. In the setting of sepsis, the use of G-CSF and GM-CSF has been studied and has not generally been found to be useful [62, 63] except in settings of prolonged neutropenia or in infants with congenital neutropenia syndromes [64].

Coagulopathy

Definition of Coagulopathy

In the neonate, the coagulation system is maturing, and levels of the various coagulation factors may not reach normal adult values for several months post birth. For this reason, simply measuring the prothrombin time (PT) or the activated partial thromboplastin time (aPTT) and comparing them to normal, adult reference ranges does not predict the bleeding risk [65, 66]. The neonatal coagulation system is dynamic and changes significantly from conception [67] until between 6 and 12 months of age when values begin to approximate adult levels for many of the coagulation parameters. This change in coagulation has been termed "developmental hemostasis" and is a careful interplay between platelet and endothelial cell function and the balance between coagulation, fibrinolysis, and natural anticoagulants (protein C and S and antithrombin). However, these differences in pro- and anticoagulant factors in the neonate/infant represent a different "set point" and do not normally predispose to either increased risk of bleeding or thrombosis. The differences in the neonate from adults are summarized in Table 3.4. Reference ranges for PT, aPTT, and the different coagulation factors for neonates therefore vary depending on gestational/postnatal age in addition to varying, to some degree, with the reagents used in the laboratory performing the testing [66, 67]. This makes assessing these parameters even more complicated in the newborn; therefore, routine testing is generally not recommended in the absence of bleeding.

Guidelines for Transfusion Practice

Currently, administration of FFP to neonates is only recommended to treat bleeding associated with coagulopathy, disseminated intravascular coagulation (DIC), and inherited deficiencies of coagulation factors when replacement products are not available [9, 68]. Routine laboratory screening of neonates for coagulopathy in the absence of bleeding is not recommended [69].

Table 3.4 Key differences between adult and neonatal hemostasis

Neonate versus older child/adult		
Primary hemostasis	Platelet function	Decreased
Coagulation factors	Vitamin K-dependent factors (II, VII, IX, X)	Decreased
	FV, FVIII	Normal or increased
	FXI	Decreased
	Fibrinogen	Normal
Natural anticoagulants	Antithrombin	Decreased
	Protein C	Decreased
	Protein S (free)	Normal or increased

Vitamin K-Deficient Bleeding: A Special Case of Coagulopathy in Neonates

In the majority of neonates, the vitamin K-dependent coagulation factors are decreased at birth. In addition, neonates are prone to vitamin K deficiency due to both low stores and relatively low intestinal colonization levels (and low ability to synthesize endogenous vitamin K) as well as poor placental transport of vitamin K combined with low concentrations in breast milk [70]. The result is that despite relatively low dietary requirements for vitamin K, neonates are at increased risk. Some neonates develop coagulopathy with deficiency of the vitamin K-dependent factors and significant bleeding symptoms. This is called vitamin K deficiency-related bleeding (VKDB) and occurs in three forms: early (within 24 h), classical (24 h–7 days), or late (2–12 weeks) [71]. The incidence of particularly late VKDB may be increasing in the USA as more parents may be choosing to refuse vitamin K prophylaxis (the routine administration of 1 mg intramuscular injection of vitamin K to prevent VKDB to all neonates at the time of delivery) [72, 73].

Early VKDB typically occurs as the result of maternal ingestion of drugs that inhibit vitamin K including anticonvulsants, antibiotics (cephalosporins and antituberculosis drugs, isoniazid and rifampin), and vitamin K antagonists. Infants often present with significant hemorrhage and manifestations can be severe [74].

Classical VKDB occurs after 24 h but within the first week of life and is generally more mild, presenting with bruising, GI blood loss, and bleeding from the umbilicus and venipuncture sites, and occurs in 1.7 % of live births without vitamin K prophylaxis [75].

Late VKDB occurs between 2 and 12 weeks postnatally and generally occurs in infants that are exclusively breastfed, in particular those infants that did not receive the vitamin K prophylaxis at birth or who have underlying impaired intestinal absorption or hepatobiliary defects [72]. The clinical presentation of late VKDB is often severe and is associated with significant mortality (14–20 %) and significant morbidity (40 % neurological morbidity) [72, 73]. This high morbidity and mortality is due to the frequency of intracranial hemorrhage occurring in 50–63 % of infants with late VKDB [76].

There are strict criteria for the definition of VKDB (because of the variability in factor levels after birth). Therefore, a confirmed case of VKDB must have a PT that is ≥4 the control value and at least one of the following:

1. Normal or increased platelet count, normal fibrinogen, and absent fibrin degradation products (i.e., no evidence of DIC).
2. PT returns to normal after vitamin K administration.
3. PIVKA (a measure of proteins produced by vitamin K absence) level exceeding that of normal controls.

Treatment of VKDB consists of subcutaneous (SQ) or intravenous (IV) vitamin K to immediately correct the deficiency and management of the bleeding symptoms. Demonstrable increases in vitamin K-dependent factors can be seen within

30 min of intravenous administration of vitamin K (1–3 mg) with normalization within 2 h [77]. Therefore, slow IV infusion is warranted in infants with bleeding. Additionally, for severe bleeding episodes, transfusion with FFP or with a prothrombin complex containing all four vitamin K-dependent factors (if available) provides immediate replacement of vitamin K-dependent factors [78].

References

1. Henry E, Christensen RD. Reference intervals in neonatal hematology. Clin Perinatol. 2015;42(3):483–97.
2. Colombatti R, Sainati L, Trevisanuto D. Anemia and transfusion in the neonate. Semin Fetal Neonatal Med. 2016;21(1):2–9.
3. Patel RM, Knezevic A, Shenvi N, Hinkes M, Keene S, Roback JD, et al. Association of Red blood cell transfusion, anemia, and necrotizing enterocolitis in very Low-birth-weight infants. JAMA. 2016;315(9):889–97.
4. Christensen RD, Carroll PD, Josephson CD. Evidence-based advances in transfusion practice in neonatal intensive care units. Neonatology. 2014;106(3):245–53.
5. Ohlsson A, Aher SM. Early erythropoietin for preventing red blood cell transfusion in preterm and/or low birth weight infants. Cochrane Database Syst Rev. 2014;4:CD004863.
6. Christensen RD, Baer VL, Lambert DK, Ilstrup SJ, Eggert LD, Henry E. Association, among very-low-birthweight neonates, between red blood cell transfusions in the week after birth and severe intraventricular hemorrhage. Transfusion. 2014;54(1):104–8.
7. Mohamed A, Shah PS. Transfusion associated necrotizing enterocolitis: a meta-analysis of observational data. Pediatrics. 2012;129(3):529–40.
8. Kasat K, Hendricks-Munoz KD, Mally PV. Neonatal red blood cell transfusions: searching for better guidelines. Blood Transfus. 2011;9(1):86–94.
9. Roseff SD, Luban NL, Manno CS. Guidelines for assessing appropriateness of pediatric transfusion. Transfusion. 2002;42(11):1398–413.
10. Girelli G, Antoncecchi S, Casadei AM, Del Vecchio A, Isernia P, Motta M, et al. Recommendations for transfusion therapy in neonatology. Blood Transfus. 2015;13(3):484–97.
11. Stevens K, Wirth FH. Incidence of neonatal hyperviscosity at sea level. J Pediatr. 1980;97(1):118–9.
12. Sarkar S, Rosenkrantz TS. Neonatal polycythemia and hyperviscosity. Semin Fetal Neonatal Med. 2008;13(4):248–55.
13. Awonusonu FO, Pauly TH, Hutchison AA. Maternal smoking and partial exchange transfusion for neonatal polycythemia. Am J Perinatol. 2002;19(7):349–54.
14. Black VD, Lubchenco LO, Koops BL, Poland RL, Powell DP. Neonatal hyperviscosity: randomized study of effect of partial plasma exchange transfusion on long-term outcome. Pediatrics. 1985;75(6):1048–53.
15. Wiswell TE, Cornish JD, Northam RS. Neonatal polycythemia: frequency of clinical manifestations and other associated findings. Pediatrics. 1986;78(1):26–30.
16. Morag I, Strauss T, Lubin D, Schushan-Eisen I, Kenet G, Kuint J. Restrictive management of neonatal polycythemia. Am J Perinatol. 2011;28(9):677–82.
17. Mimouni FB, Merlob P, Dollberg S, Mandel D, Israeli Neonatal A. Neonatal polycythaemia: critical review and a consensus statement of the Israeli Neonatology Association. Acta Paediatr. 2011;100(10):1290–6.
18. Watchko JF. Common hematologic problems in the newborn nursery. Pediatr Clin North Am. 2015;62(2):509–24.

19. Cremer M, Sallmon H, Kling PJ, Buhrer C, Dame C. Thrombocytopenia and platelet transfusion in the neonate. Semin Fetal Neonatal Med. 2016;21(1):10–8.
20. Bussel JB, Berkowitz RL, Hung C, Kolb EA, Wissert M, Primiani A, et al. Intracranial hemorrhage in alloimmune thrombocytopenia: stratified management to prevent recurrence in the subsequent affected fetus. Am J Obstet Gynecol. 2010;203(2):135.e1–14.
21. Tiller H, Killie MK, Skogen B, Oian P, Husebekk A. Neonatal alloimmune thrombocytopenia in Norway: poor detection rate with nonscreening versus a general screening programme. BJOG. 2009;116(4):594–8.
22. Mueller-Eckhardt C, Kiefel V, Grubert A, Kroll H, Weisheit M, Schmidt S, et al. 348 cases of suspected neonatal alloimmune thrombocytopenia. Lancet. 1989;1(8634):363–6.
23. Bussel JB, Zabusky MR, Berkowitz RL, McFarland JG. Fetal alloimmune thrombocytopenia. N Engl J Med. 1997;337(1):22–6.
24. Lewin S, Bussel JB. Review of fetal and neonatal immune cytopenias. Clin Adv Hematol Oncol. 2015;13(1):35–43.
25. Bussel JB, Sola-Visner M. Current approaches to the evaluation and management of the fetus and neonate with immune thrombocytopenia. Semin Perinatol. 2009;33(1):35–42.
26. Williamson LM, Hackett G, Rennie J, Palmer CR, Maciver C, Hadfield R, et al. The natural history of fetomaternal alloimmunization to the platelet-specific antigen HPA-1a (PlA1, Zwa) as determined by antenatal screening. Blood. 1998;92(7):2280–7.
27. Vadasz B, Zdravic PC, Li J, Li C, Carri N, Ni H. Platelets and platelet alloantigens: lessons from human patients and animal models of fetal and neonatal alloimmune thrombocytopenia. Genes Dis. 2015;2(2):173–85.
28. Bussel JB, Primiani A. Fetal and neonatal alloimmune thrombocytopenia: progress and ongoing debates. Blood Rev. 2008;22(1):33–52.
29. Ouwehand WH, Smith G, Ranasinghe E. Management of severe alloimmune thrombocytopenia in the newborn. Arch Dis Child Fetal Neonatal Ed. 2000;82(3):F173–5.
30. Bakchoul T, Bassler D, Heckmann M, Thiele T, Kiefel V, Gross I, et al. Management of infants born with severe neonatal alloimmune thrombocytopenia: the role of platelet transfusions and intravenous immunoglobulin. Transfusion. 2014;54(3):640–5.
31. McQuilten ZK, Wood EM, Savoia H, Cole S. A review of pathophysiology and current treatment for neonatal alloimmune thrombocytopenia (NAIT) and introducing the Australian NAIT registry. Aust N Z J Obstet Gynaecol. 2011;51(3):191–8.
32. Peterson JA, McFarland JG, Curtis BR, Aster RH. Neonatal alloimmune thrombocytopenia: pathogenesis, diagnosis and management. Br J Haematol. 2013;161(1):3–14.
33. van der Lugt NM, van Kampen A, Walther FJ, Brand A, Lopriore E. Outcome and management in neonatal thrombocytopenia due to maternal idiopathic thrombocytopenic purpura. Vox Sang. 2013;105(3):236–43.
34. Fujimura K, Harada Y, Fujimoto T, Kuramoto A, Ikeda Y, Akatsuka J, et al. Nationwide study of idiopathic thrombocytopenic purpura in pregnant women and the clinical influence on neonates. Int J Hematol. 2002;75(4):426–33.
35. Koyama S, Tomimatsu T, Kanagawa T, Kumasawa K, Tsutsui T, Kimura T. Reliable predictors of neonatal immune thrombocytopenia in pregnant women with idiopathic thrombocytopenic purpura. Am J Hematol. 2012;87(1):15–21.
36. Christiaens GC, Nieuwenhuis HK, Bussel JB. Comparison of platelet counts in first and second newborns of mothers with immune thrombocytopenic purpura. Obstet Gynecol. 1997;90(4 Pt 1):546–52.
37. Payne SD, Resnik R, Moore TR, Hedriana HL, Kelly TF. Maternal characteristics and risk of severe neonatal thrombocytopenia and intracranial hemorrhage in pregnancies complicated by autoimmune thrombocytopenia. Am J Obstet Gynecol. 1997;177(1):149–55.
38. Stanworth SJ. Thrombocytopenia, bleeding, and use of platelet transfusions in sick neonates. Hematol Am Soc Hematol Educ Program. 2012;2012:512–6.
39. Hohlfeld P, Forestier F, Kaplan C, Tissot JD, Daffos F. Fetal thrombocytopenia: a retrospective survey of 5,194 fetal blood samplings. Blood. 1994;84(6):1851–6.

40. Stanworth SJ, Clarke P, Watts T, Ballard S, Choo L, Morris T, et al. Prospective, observational study of outcomes in neonates with severe thrombocytopenia. Pediatrics. 2009;124(5):e826–34.
41. Curley A, Venkatesh V, Stanworth S, Clarke P, Watts T, New H, et al. Platelets for neonatal transfusion: study 2 – a randomised controlled trial to compare two different platelet count thresholds for prophylactic platelet transfusion to preterm neonates. Neonatology. 2014;106(2):102–6.
42. Venkatesh V, Curley AE, Clarke P, Watts T, Stanworth SJ. Do we know when to treat neonatal thrombocytopaenia? Arch Dis Child Fetal Neonatal Ed. 2013;98(5):F380–2.
43. Murray NA, Howarth LJ, McCloy MP, Letsky EA, Roberts IA. Platelet transfusion in the management of severe thrombocytopenia in neonatal intensive care unit patients. Transfus Med. 2002;12(1):35–41.
44. von Lindern JS, Hulzebos CV, Bos AF, Brand A, Walther FJ, Lopriore E. Thrombocytopaenia and intraventricular haemorrhage in very premature infants: a tale of two cities. Arch Dis Child Fetal Neonatal Ed. 2012;97(5):F348–52.
45. Josephson CD, Su LL, Christensen RD, Hillyer CD, Castillejo MI, Emory MR, et al. Platelet transfusion practices among neonatologists in the United States and Canada: results of a survey. Pediatrics. 2009;123(1):278–85.
46. Baley JE, Stork EK, Warkentin PI, Shurin SB. Neonatal neutropenia. Clinical manifestations, cause, and outcome. Am J Dis Child. 1988;142(11):1161–6.
47. al-Mulla ZS, Christensen RD. Neutropenia in the neonate. Clin Perinatol. 1995;22(3):711–39.
48. Maheshwari A. Neutropenia in the newborn. Curr Opin Hematol. 2014;21(1):43–9.
49. Gray PH, Rodwell RL. Neonatal neutropenia associated with maternal hypertension poses a risk for nosocomial infection. Eur J Pediatr. 1999;158(1):71–3.
50. Cartron J, Tchernia G, Celton JL, Damay M, Cheron G, Farrokhi P, et al. Alloimmune neonatal neutropenia. Am J Pediatr Hematol Oncol. 1991;13(1):21–5.
51. Funke A, Berner R, Traichel B, Schmeisser D, Leititis JU, Niemeyer CM. Frequency, natural course, and outcome of neonatal neutropenia. Pediatrics. 2000;106(1 Pt 1):45–51.
52. Koenig JM, Christensen RD. Incidence, neutrophil kinetics, and natural history of neonatal neutropenia associated with maternal hypertension. N Engl J Med. 1989;321(9):557–62.
53. Manzoni P. Hematologic aspects of early and late-onset sepsis in preterm infants. Clin Perinatol. 2015;42(3):587–95.
54. Farruggia P. Immune neutropenias of infancy and childhood. World J Pediatr. 2016;12(2):142–8.
55. Christensen RD, Calhoun DA, Rimsza LM. A practical approach to evaluating and treating neutropenia in the neonatal intensive care unit. Clin Perinatol. 2000;27(3):577–601.
56. van den Tooren-de Groot R, Ottink M, Huiskes E, van Rossum A, van der Voorn B, Slomp J, et al. Management and outcome of 35 cases with foetal/neonatal alloimmune neutropenia. Acta Paediatr. 2014;103(11):e467–74.
57. Zupanska B, Uhrynowska M, Guz K, Maslanka K, Brojer E, Czestynska M, et al. The risk of antibody formation against HNA1a and HNA1b granulocyte antigens during pregnancy and its relation to neonatal neutropenia. Transfus Med. 2001;11(5):377–82.
58. Bux J, Jung KD, Kauth T, Mueller-Eckhardt C. Serological and clinical aspects of granulocyte antibodies leading to alloimmune neonatal neutropenia. Transfus Med. 1992;2(2):143–9.
59. Bux J, Behrens G, Jaeger G, Welte K. Diagnosis and clinical course of autoimmune neutropenia in infancy: analysis of 240 cases. Blood. 1998;91(1):181–6.
60. Rodwell RL, Gray PH, Taylor KM, Minchinton R. Granulocyte colony stimulating factor treatment for alloimmune neonatal neutropenia. Arch Dis Child Fetal Neonatal Ed. 1996;75(1):F57–8.
61. Mohan P, Brocklehurst P. Granulocyte transfusions for neonates with confirmed or suspected sepsis and neutropaenia. Cochrane Database Syst Rev. 2003(4):CD003956.

62. Bernstein HM, Pollock BH, Calhoun DA, Christensen RD. Administration of recombinant granulocyte colony-stimulating factor to neonates with septicemia: a meta-analysis. J Pediatr. 2001;138(6):917–20.

63. Carr R, Modi N, Dore C. G-CSF and GM-CSF for treating or preventing neonatal infections. Cochrane Database Syst Rev. 2003(3):CD003066.

64. Dale DC, Cottle TE, Fier CJ, Bolyard AA, Bonilla MA, Boxer LA, et al. Severe chronic neutropenia: treatment and follow-up of patients in the Severe Chronic Neutropenia International Registry. Am J Hematol. 2003;72(2):82–93.

65. Andrew M, Paes B, Milner R, Johnston M, Mitchell L, Tollefsen DM, et al. Development of the human coagulation system in the full-term infant. Blood. 1987;70(1):165–72.

66. Andrew M, Paes B, Milner R, Johnston M, Mitchell L, Tollefsen DM, et al. Development of the human coagulation system in the healthy premature infant. Blood. 1988;72(5):1651–7.

67. Christensen RD, Baer VL, Lambert DK, Henry E, Ilstrup SJ, Bennett ST. Reference intervals for common coagulation tests of preterm infants (CME). Transfusion. 2014;54(3):627–32; quiz 6.

68. Motta M, Testa M, Tripodi G, Radicioni M. Changes in neonatal transfusion practice after dissemination of neonatal recommendations. Pediatrics. 2010;125(4):e810–7.

69. Motta M, Del Vecchio A, Perrone B, Ghirardello S, Radicioni M. Fresh frozen plasma use in the NICU: a prospective, observational, multicentred study. Arch Dis Child Fetal Neonatal Ed. 2014;99(4):F303–8.

70. Van Winckel M, De Bruyne R, Van De Velde S, Van Biervliet S. Vitamin K, an update for the paediatrician. Eur J Pediatr. 2009;168(2):127–34.

71. Lippi G, Franchini M. Vitamin K in neonates: facts and myths. Blood Transfus. 2011;9(1):4–9.

72. Schulte R, Jordan LC, Morad A, Naftel RP, Wellons 3rd JC, Sidonio R. Rise in late onset vitamin K deficiency bleeding in young infants because of omission or refusal of prophylaxis at birth. Pediatr Neurol. 2014;50(6):564–8.

73. Centers for Disease C, Prevention. Notes from the field: late vitamin K deficiency bleeding in infants whose parents declined vitamin K prophylaxis – Tennessee, 2013. MMWR Morb Mortal Wkly Rep. 2013;62(45):901–2.

74. Pichler E, Pichler L. The neonatal coagulation system and the vitamin K deficiency bleeding: a mini review. Wien Med Wochenschr. 2008;158(13–14):385–95.

75. American Academy of Pediatrics Committee on F, Newborn. Controversies concerning vitamin K and the newborn. American Academy of Pediatrics Committee on Fetus and Newborn. Pediatrics. 2003;112(1 Pt 1):191–2.

76. Loughnan PM, McDougall PN. Epidemiology of late onset haemorrhagic disease: a pooled data analysis. J Paediatr Child Health. 1993;29(3):177–81.

77. Shearer MJ. Vitamin K, deficiency bleeding (VKDB) in early infancy. Blood Rev. 2009;23(2):49–59.

78. O'Shaughnessy DF, Atterbury C, Bolton Maggs P, Murphy M, Thomas D, Yates S, et al. Guidelines for the use of fresh-frozen plasma, cryoprecipitate and cryosupernatant. Br J Haematol. 2004;126(1):11–28.

Chapter 4
Hemolytic Disease of the Fetus and Newborn

Sara C. Handley and Michael A. Posencheg

Diagnosis

Hemolytic disease of the fetus and newborn (HDFN) is a group of disorders that result in progressive hyperbilirubinemia and anemia, with or without the presence of edema, in the fetus or newborn. This disease was previously synonymous with hemolytic disease resulting from Rh isoimmunization. With the onset of the use of Rh immunoglobulin (RhIG) in pregnant Rh-negative women approximately 45 years ago, the landscape of this disorder has changed dramatically. The differential diagnosis of hemolytic disease of the fetus and newborn (HDFN) is broad and can be subdivided into isoimmune and nonimmune categories (See Table 4.1). In this chapter, we will review various diseases that result in fetal and neonatal hemolysis, recent improvements in diagnosis and management, and requirements for exchange transfusions in certain circumstances.

Isoimmune hemolytic disease in the fetus and newborn manifests when maternal IgG antibodies cross the placenta and bind to antigens present on fetal/newborn red blood cells. Red cell destruction results when the antibody-coated cells are scavenged by the mononuclear phagocytic system. The major categories of antigens include Rh factor (e.g., D antigen), leading to Rh isoimmunization, the major blood group antigens (e.g., A or B) leading to ABO incompatibility, and minor blood group antigens (e.g., Kell, Kidd, or Duffy). The incidence of Rh isoimmunization

S.C. Handley, MD
Department of Pediatrics, The Children's Hospital of Philadelphia,
3401 Civic Center Blvd, Philadelphia, PA 19104, USA
e-mail: handleys@email.chop.edu

M.A. Posencheg, MD (✉)
Neonatology and Newborn Services, Hospital of the University of Pennsylvania,
Perelman School of Medicine University of Pennsylvania, 3400 Spruce Street,
Ravdin Building, 8th Floor, Philadelphia, PA 19104, USA
e-mail: Michael.posencheg@uphs.upenn.edu

© Springer International Publishing Switzerland 2017
D.A. Sesok-Pizzini (ed.), *Neonatal Transfusion Practices*,
DOI 10.1007/978-3-319-42764-5_4

Table 4.1 Causes of hemolytic disease of the fetus and newborn

Isoimmune hemolysis	Nonimmune mediated
Rh isoimmunization	RBC membrane disorders (e.g., hereditary spherocytosis)
ABO incompatibility	RBC enzyme defects (e.g., G6PD deficiency)
Antibody-mediated hemolysis due to minor antigens	Hemoglobinopathies (e.g., alpha-thalassemia)

has fallen from nearly 14 % of pregnancies in the pre-RhIG era to between 1 and 6 per 1000 live births. Incomplete eradication is due to inadvertent failures of RhIG administration, poor prenatal care, or earlier sensitization [1]. Rh isoimmunization can lead to severe complications with up to 20 % of fetuses having significant anemia and evidence of hydrops fetalis in utero.

ABO incompatibility occurs nearly exclusively in fetuses and newborns with type A or B blood born to mothers with type O blood. While approximately 15 % of pregnancies result in a mismatch of maternal (type O) and neonatal (type A or B) blood, about a third of these have a positive direct antiglobulin or Coombs' test (DAT). Furthermore, only 15–50 % of infants with a positive DAT demonstrate significant hemolytic disease as evidenced by a peak total serum bilirubin (TSB) level over 12.8 mg/dl or an hour-specific TSB >95 % on the Bhutani nomogram. Therefore, clinically significant disease occurs in only 1–5 % of infants born to mothers with type O blood [2]. In the rare occurrence when ABO incompatibility has been seen in an A–B maternal–infant mismatch, it has been associated with an extraordinarily high anti-B IgG antibody titer [3]. Lastly, in contrast to HDFN resulting from either Rh isoimmunization or from minor group antibodies, hemolytic disease in maternal–infant pairs with ABO incompatibility can occur in first pregnancies. IgG to both the A and B antigens are naturally occurring and do not require prior sensitization to be produced.

The incidence of hemolytic disease from minor antigens is more difficult to estimate due to the large number of antigen–antibody reactions that can result in disease. Of the minor antigens, Kell (anti-K) and Duffy (anti-Fy^a) antigens are associated with the most severe disease, while Lewis and Lutheran are more likely associated with mild or insignificant hemolysis. Table 4.2 provides a summary of a selection of these antibodies and their potential impact on the fetus or newborn [1, 4].

The group of disorders that are nonimmune in nature result in red blood cell destruction in the absence of an antibody–antigen reaction. These include red blood cell membrane defects such as hereditary elliptocytosis or spherocytosis, red blood cell enzyme defects such as glucose-6-phosphate dehydrogenase (G6PD) deficiency and pyruvate kinase deficiency, and hemoglobinopathies such as alpha-thalassemia. With rates up to 1 in 1000–2000 live births, hereditary spherocytosis is the most common of the RBC membrane defects, occurring most commonly in infants of Northern European descent [5]. Of the enzyme defects, G6PD is the most common, especially in infants of African or Mediterranean descent. It is an X-linked disorder

Table 4.2 Selected minor antigens associated with fetal or neonatal hemolytic disease

Blood group	Severe disease	Rarely severe disease	Mild disease	Usually no disease
Rh	D, c	C, E, f, Evans, G, Rh29, Rh32, Rh42, Rh46, and others	E, e, f	
Lutheran			Lu^a, Lu^b	
Kell	K	k, Kp^a, Kp^b, Ku, Js^a, Js^b, K11, K22	Ku, Js^a, K11	K23, K24
Lewis				Le^a, Le^b
Duffy		Fy^a	Fy^b, Fy3	
Kidd		Jk^a	Jk^b, Jk3	

Adapted from Eder [1] and Moise [4]

that is most commonly seen in male infants; however, females can also manifest the disease. Interestingly, this disease accounts for a disproportionately large percentage of infants who develop kernicterus, especially among African-Americans [6]. Alpha-thalassemia, in its most severe form, is a rare hemoglobinopathy in which all alpha-globin chain genes are deleted. It is most common in Asian infants and is nearly uniformly fatal with severe fetal anemia and hydrops fetalis, especially when intrauterine transfusions have not been performed.

In the neonate, concern for hemolytic anemia results from one or more of the following clinical conditions: a rapidly rising bilirubin level, especially in the first 24 hours of life, a positive direct Coombs' test, hemolysis detected on a blood smear with anemia detected on a complete blood count (CBC), or prolonged hyperbilirubinemia. In addition to following serial bilirubin levels, in this setting the practitioner should include a neonatal blood type, Coombs' (DAT) test, and complete blood count with reticulocyte count to determine whether hemolysis is occurring.

In general, the presence of a positive DAT in the appropriate clinical setting suggests isoimmune hemolysis, while a negative DAT nearly rules it out. There are rare instances of isoimmune hemolysis with a false-negative DAT. Interestingly, infants can have a positive Coombs' test and not have clinically significant hemolysis. In this situation, obtaining a CBC and a reticulocyte count can be helpful in determining which infants are experiencing hemolysis. Due to high erythropoietin levels just before birth, a newborn in the first day or two of life can have a reticulocyte count of up to approximately 7 % and be considered normal. This returns to a baseline of 1–2 % by approximately 4 days of life.

A G6PD level can also be helpful in establishing a diagnosis in infants with the appropriate ethnic background or geographical distribution. Many states have adopted universal newborn screening for G6PD deficiency. Furthermore, serum albumin, the primary protein transporter for bilirubin in the blood, can also be measured. Low serum levels of albumin increase the risk of developing neurological sequelae from the subsequent increased amount of free, unbound bilirubin crossing the blood–brain barrier.

Treatment Including Exchange Transfusions

The goals of therapy are different depending on the timing of disease. When significant hemolysis occurs in utero, the fetus becomes progressively anemic. In the fetus, bilirubin is normally processed and excreted through the placenta. Therefore, the primary concern is to treat the anemia and, in doing so, prevent or reverse any signs of edema or hydrops fetalis. In this circumstance, percutaneous umbilical blood sampling (PUBS) and intrauterine blood transfusion can diagnose and treat fetal anemia, respectively. In general, intrauterine transfusions are performed from approximately 20–35 weeks gestation when the fetal hematocrit falls to 25–30 % [7].

In the neonate, the problem is somewhat different. In the absence of placental transfer and maternal clearance of bilirubin, the neonate must now take on this task. However, in the first days of life, infants are ill equipped to do so due to inadequate activity of the glucuronyl-transferase enzyme that conjugates bilirubin produced from the high heme load resulting from significant hemolysis. This leads to accumulation of bilirubin because it must be conjugated to be excreted. Therefore, the more pressing problem faced by the pediatrician is often the hyperbilirubinemia. The mainstay for treatment of hyperbilirubinemia is phototherapy. Figure 4.1 contains the phototherapy treatment guidelines for infants greater than or equal to 35 weeks gestation as published by the American Academy of Pediatrics (AAP) in 2004 [8]. To use the chart, the practitioner must know the gestational age of the

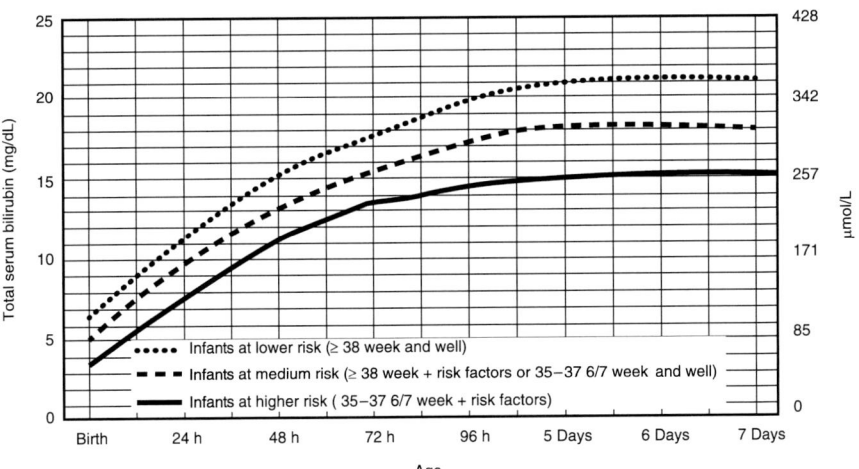

- Use total bilirubin. Do not subtract direct reacting or conjugated bilirubin.
- Risk factors a isoimmune hemolytic disease, G6PD deficiency, asphyxia, significant lethargy, temperature instability. sepsis, acidosis, or albumin < 3.0 g/dL (if measured)
- For well infants 35–37 6/7 week can adjust TSB levels for intervention around the medium risk line It is an option to intervene at lower TSB levels for infants closer to 35 weeks and at higher TSB levels for those closer to 37 6/7 week.
- It is an option to provice conventional phototherapy in hospital or at home at TSB levels 2–3 mg/dL (35–50 mmol/L) below those shown out home phototherapy should not be used in any infant with risk factors.

Fig. 4.1 Hour-specific treatment nomogram for phototherapy (From American Academy of Pediatrics, 2004)

infant, hours of life, and the presence or absence of risk factors associated with neurological complications. It is important to know that isoimmune hemolytic disease is considered one of these risk factors.

Unconjugated bilirubin absorbs light maximally in the blue portion of the visible spectrum (approximately 450 nm). Phototherapy with a light source that approximates this spectrum results in the photoisomerization of unconjugated bilirubin into a polar, water-soluble, and more readily excretable form. As a result, both configurational and structural isomers are formed; the most common structural isomer is called lumirubin. The efficacy of phototherapy is related to the spectrum of light used, irradiance of light, exposed surface area of the skin, and distance of light source from the infant.

In the setting of isoimmune (or antibody-associated) hemolysis, the use of intravenous immune globulin (IVIG) has been shown to decrease the need for exchange transfusion and is a helpful adjunctive therapy. The current recommendation from the American Academy of Pediatrics (AAP) is to administer IVIG 0.5–1 g/kg over 2 hours if the total serum bilirubin (TSB) is rising despite phototherapy or if the TSB is within 2–3 mg/dl of the exchange transfusion level. This dose can be repeated in 12 hours [8].

For some infants, the use of phototherapy and IVIG, if indicated, is not sufficient to control the rising bilirubin level. Alternatively, some infants may have neurological manifestations of bilirubin toxicity despite bilirubin levels below suggested therapeutic levels. In these instances, a double volume exchange transfusion (DVET) is indicated. This procedure involves the removal of twice the infant's blood volume with simultaneous isovolemic replacement of reconstituted whole blood. This process achieves two separate but related goals. First, it removes bilirubin, and, second, in the setting of isoimmune hemolytic disease, it removes offending maternal antibodies. While criteria to perform a DVET is clearly outlined in the guidelines from the AAP published in 2004 and shown in Fig. 4.2, some experts suggest performing a DVET at even lower levels when significant antibody-mediated hemolysis is occurring due to the added benefit provided by removing maternal antibodies. Furthermore, the presence of isoimmune hemolytic disease lowers the threshold for which a DVET is indicated due to the increased risk of kernicterus in this setting [8].

Prevention

The administration of Rh immunoglobulin (RhIG) to mothers who are Rh negative has dramatically decreased the incidence of hemolytic disease resulting from Rh isoimmunization. The current recommendations of the American College of Obstetrics and Gynecology (ACOG) are to administer 300 μg of RhIG intramuscularly at 28 weeks gestation and within 72 h of delivery of an Rh-positive infant to an Rh-negative mother. Furthermore, RhIG should also be administered to Rh-negative mothers if one of the following events occur: amniocentesis, chorionic villus sampling, cordocentesis, abdominal trauma, external cephalic version, or maternal bleeding due to

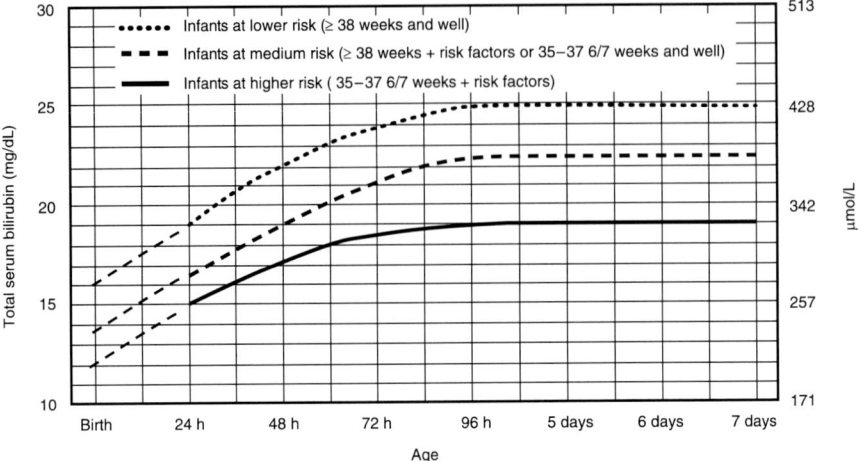

- The dashed lines for the first 24 h indicate uncertainty due to a wide range of clinical circumstances and a range of responses to phototherapy.
- Immediate exchange transfusion is recommended if infant shows signs of acute bilirubin encephalopathy (hypertonia, arching, retrocollis, opisthotonos, fever, high pitched cry) or if TSB is ≥5 mg/dL (85μmol/L) above these lines.
- Risk factors – isoimmune hemolytic disease, GBPD deficiency, asphyxia, significant lethargy, temperature instability. sepsis, acidosis
- Measure serum albumin and calculate B/A ratio (See legend)
- Use total bilirubin. Do not subtract direct reacting or conjugated bilirubin.
- If infant is well and 35–37 6/7 weeks (median risk) can individualize TSB evels for exchange based on actual gestational age.

Fig. 4.2 Hour-specific treatment nomogram for double volume exchange transfusion (From American Academy of Pediatrics, 2004)

placental abruption, placenta previa, partial molar pregnancy, spontaneous abortion, or elective termination [9]. Controversy exists regarding the use of RhIG in the first trimester. As early as 7 weeks of gestation, fetal blood cells can express the D antigen, and women with threatened abortion in the first trimester have been shown to become Rh sensitized, although this is rare event. Some advocate for administration of RhIG 50 μg intramuscularly in the first trimester in the setting of spontaneous abortion, elective termination, ectopic pregnancy, or threatened abortion. The proposed mechanism of action for RhIG involves binding to Rh-positive fetal cells with resultant scavenging by the maternal mononuclear phagocytic system prior to sensitization and production of maternal antibody against the Rh-D antigen. Sadly, the other forms of hemolytic disease do not have specific preventative strategies.

Monitoring

Monitoring of hemolytic anemia can be performed in utero and after delivery. Significant advances have improved our ability to determine the degree of fetal anemia using both invasive and noninvasive studies. Routine screening performed early in gestation includes maternal blood type, Rh status, and antibody screening. Antibody screening, using an indirect Coombs' test, can identify the presence of antibodies directed against fetal red blood cells. If the test is positive, the antibody is subsequently typed and titers obtained. Maternal antibody titers are monitored during pregnancy, until the critical titer threshold is reached. The critical threshold may vary by institution, methodology, and antibody type; however, most centers consider a titer of 1:16 or 1:32 suggestive of significant hemolysis risk.

Some centers employ further testing, including paternal antigen testing to determine paternal Rh status, which can help inform fetal risk and monitoring needs. If appropriate, an amniocentesis can be performed to determine fetal blood type if a critical titer, as described above, has been reached. Cell-free fetal DNA, a significantly less invasive test to determine fetal Rh status, has shown accurate prediction in 99.5% of cases, and some laboratories can also determine fetal Kell, C, c and E antibody status [10]. However, this testing approach is not yet standard of care.

Liley first described the relationship between bilirubin level in the amniotic fluid and the degree of fetal anemia in infants greater than 27 weeks gestation [11]. In this method, an amniocentesis is performed, and amniotic fluid is analyzed at a wavelength of 450 nm (ΔOD_{450}) to determine the bilirubin level; the resulting value is plotted on validated graphs to assess risk. Interventions including delivery or intrauterine transfusion are suggested if the level is above a specified threshold. An expanded form of the Liley curve, as well as the development of the Queenan curve, has provided practitioners with improved, yet still invasive, tools to determine the risk of Rh isoimmune fetal anemia as early as 14 weeks gestation [12]. However, these methods may be less useful when antibodies to the Kell antigens are involved.

A noninvasive and generally preferred option for assessing the severity of fetal anemia is the measurement of middle cerebral artery peak systolic velocity (MCA-PSV) by Doppler ultrasonography. Theoretically, as a fetus becomes more anemic and compensates to preserve oxygen delivery, the cerebral blood flow velocity increases due to increased cardiac output and vasodilatation, resulting in an increased MCA-PSV. The measurement is gestational age specific, and a value greater than 1.5 multiples of the median (MoM) suggests moderate to severe anemia with a sensitivity of 88–100% [13, 14]. The effect of intrauterine transfusions on this measurement is unclear, as the presence of adult red blood cells may alter the interpretation of MCA-PSV. A large, prospective, randomized multicenter study compared the use of ΔOD_{450} to MCA-PSV and found that MCA Dopplers were more sensitive (88% versus 76%), but less specific than $\Delta OD\ 450$ (82% versus 77%) [15].

The gold standard for measuring fetal anemia is fetal blood sampling via the umbilical vein, which may be referred to as cordocentesis, funipuncture, or percutaneous umbilical blood sampling (PUBS). In addition to determining the level of anemia, fetal blood type, Coombs' testing, reticulocyte count, and total bilirubin can be determined if appropriate. However, this procedure carries significant risks, including cord bleeding and hematomas, fetal bradycardia, infection, placental abruption, further maternal sensitization from fetomaternal hemorrhage, and fetal/perinatal death. If a fetus' hematocrit is two standard deviations below the mean for gestational age, an intrauterine intravascular fetal transfusion may be considered, a procedure that is technically similar to fetal blood sampling and is associated with similar risks [16]. Infants with moderate to severe anemia often require preterm delivery.

After birth, neonates at risk for hemolytic anemia must be monitored for the degree of anemia and for development of significant hyperbilirubinemia. Many institutions also determine neonatal blood type and direct antiglobulin test (DAT) status after delivery in infants who are thought to be at increased risk for hemolytic disease (specifically, those born to mothers with blood type O). However, large studies have failed to justify this approach given the cost and weak positive predictive value of DAT [17]. In the 2004 AAP position statement, this approach is not currently recommended.

In utero, bilirubin is transferred to the maternal circulation via the placenta and processed in the maternal liver, which explains why hyperbilirubinemia is a postnatal event. Early and frequent bilirubin levels and complete blood counts allow the practitioner to determine if intervention is required. The availability of hour-specific nomograms describing the risk of severe hyperbilirubinemia based on the level of bilirubin can be used in term infants to guide appropriate therapy (such as phototherapy or double volume exchange transfusion) and the timing of outpatient follow-up. These nomograms are published in the AAP position statement from 2004 as well as a subsequent clarifying publication in 2009 [8, 18]. See Figs. 4.1 and 4.2 for the phototherapy and DVET treatment nomograms for infants greater than or equal to 35 weeks gestation.

Transfusion Requirements

A double volume exchange transfusion (DVET) involves the removal and replacement of approximately twice the infant's blood volume. As described above, the indication and threshold for this procedure is based on significant hyperbilirubinemia as described in the 2004 AAP position statement. Of note, there have been studies of both packed red blood cell (PRBC) transfusion and single volume exchange transfusion for isoimmune hemolysis; however, there is inadequate evidence to support either of these interventions as the standard of care [19, 20].

Either stored whole blood or reconstituted whole blood can be used to perform an exchange transfusion with no significant differences in post DVET lab values or complications [21]. The advantage of using reconstituted whole blood allows the treatment to be tailored to the specific clinical condition, which is especially important in antibody-mediated isoimmune hemolytic disease. Depending on the offending antibody, the appropriate blood type, Rh status, and minor antigens of the cells can be selected and matched. Additionally, the plasma can be chosen to minimize subsequent hemolysis (using AB plasma or plasma compatible to the mother and neonate's serum). Blood for exchange transfusion should be washed or leuko-reduced and, ideally, irradiated to reduce the risk of transfusion reaction. The hematocrit of the reconstituted blood for DVET should be between 40 and 60%. This is obtained by diluting the RBCs with the appropriate amount of plasma.

The estimated blood volume of a term infant is 80 ml/kg; of a preterm infant, it is 100 ml/kg. The equation to determine the amount of whole/reconstituted blood needed for a DVET is as follows: estimated total blood volume (either term or preterm in ml/kg) × weight (kg) × 2 + 50–100 ml (required for priming, exact volume is institution dependent). Prior to use, the blood must be warmed using a blood warmer. The removal and infusion of blood must be done slowly, especially in ill or hemodynamically unstable infants, to minimize further hemodynamic changes. Aliquots are withdrawn slowly, though there is some variation on recommended rates and volumes. The formula 2 ml/kg/min × weight (kg) × length of pass (5 min) has been recommended to determine the appropriate aliquot for withdrawal (formula from our local DVET protocol). Others recommend removal of no more than 5 ml/kg per aliquot. If the infant does not tolerate the procedure, smaller aliquots (1 ml/kg/min × weight (kg) × length of pass) can be utilized.

Many units have developed standardized procedures for DVET, outlining appropriate access, equipment, clinical monitoring, and interval laboratory assessments. Access options, in order of preference, include an umbilical arterial catheter (for withdrawal) and an umbilical venous catheter (for transfusion), an umbilical arterial catheter (for withdrawal) and a peripheral vein (for transfusion), or an umbilical venous catheter (for both withdrawal and transfusion). If umbilical access cannot be obtained, a peripheral arterial line (for withdrawal) and a peripheral vein (for transfusion) can be used. Location of catheters should be confirmed prior to the procedure. Given presumed changes in intestinal blood flow in infants during DVET, it is often recommended that infants are NPO for at least 4 hours prior to the procedure. Prior to the procedure, a baseline complete blood count, reticulocyte count, basic metabolic panel, and blood gas with ionized calcium should be obtained. The newborn screen and other labs impacted by blood transfusions should also be collected. During the DVET, glucose levels and blood gases with ionized calcium should continue to be monitored, given the risk for hypocalcemia. Repeat pre-procedure labs should be obtained after completion of the DVET and a follow-up complete blood count and bilirubin obtained four hours after completion.

Double volume exchange transfusion carries both peri- and post-procedure risks. Periprocedure hemodynamic instability and arrhythmias have been reported. After a DVET, coagulopathy, specifically thrombocytopenia, is relatively common as neither whole nor reconstituted blood contains platelets; however, intervention including platelet transfusion is rarely needed. Additional complications may include electrolyte imbalances, infection, necrotizing enterocolitis, and death. However, these are all exceedingly rare. Continued assessment of both bilirubin and hemoglobin levels are required, as some patients require a second DVET, since the first procedure only removed approximately 86% of the infant's blood and less than 50% of bilirubin.

References

1. Eder AF. Update on HDFN: new information on long-standing controversies. Immunohematology. 2006;22(4):188–95.
2. Watchko JF. Common hematologic problems in the newborn nursery. Pediatr Clin N Am. 2015;62:509–24.
3. Wang M, Hays T, Ambruso D, Silliman C. Hemolytic disease of the newborn caused by a high titer anti-group B IgG from a group A mother. Pediatr Blood Cancer. 2005;45:861–2.
4. Moise KJ. Fetal anemia due to non-Rhesus-D red-cell alloimmunization. Semin Fetal Neonatal Med. 2008;13:207–14.
5. Christensen R, Yaish H, Gallagher P. A pediatrican's practical guide to diagnosing and treating hereditary spherocytosis in neonates. Pediatrics. 2015;135(6):1107–14.
6. Johnson L, Bhutani VK, Karp K, et al. Clinical report from the pilot USA Kernicterus Registry (1992–2004). J Perinatol. 2009;29(S1):S25–45.
7. Moise KJ. Red blood cell administration in pregnancy. Semin Hematol. 2005;42:169–78.
8. American Academy of Pediatrics. Subcommittee on hyperbilirubinemia: management of hyperbilirubinemia in the newborn infant 35 or more weeks of gestation. Pediatrics. 2004;114(1):297–316.
9. American College of Obstetricians and Gynecologists, Prevention of RhD alloimmunization. ACOG Practice Bulletin Number 4. Washington, DC; 1999.
10. Geifman-Holtzman O, Grotegut C, Gaughan J. Diagnostic accuracy of noninvasive fetal Rh genotyping from maternal blood: a meta-analysis. Am J Obstet Gynecol. 2006;195(4):1163–73.
11. Liley A. Liquor amnil analysis in the management of the pregnancy complicated by resus sensitization. Am J Obstet Gynecol. 1961;82:1359–70.
12. Queenan J, Tomai T, Ural S, King J. Deviation in amniotic fluid optical density at a wavelength of 450 nm in Rh-immunized pregnancies from 14 to 40 weeks' gestation: a proposal for clinical management. Am J Obstet Gynecol. 1993;168(5):1370–6.
13. Zimmerman R, Carpenter R, Durig P, Mari G. Longitudinal measurement of peak systolic velocity in the fetal middle cerebral artery for monitoring pregnancies complicated by red cell alloimmunisation: a prospective multicentre trial with intention-to-treat. BJOG. 2002;109(7):746–52.
14. Mari G, Hanif F. Fetal Doppler: umbilical artery, middle cerebral artery, and venous system. Semin Perinatol. 2008;32(4):253–7.
15. Oepkes D, Seaward P, Vandenbussche F, et al. Doppler ultrasonography versus amniocentesis to predict fetal anemia. N Engl J Med. 2006;355(2):156–64.
16. Van Kamp I, Klumper F, Oepkes D, et al. Complications of intrauterine intravascular transfusion for fetal anemia due to maternal red-cell alloimmunization. Am J Obstet Gynecol. 2005;192(1):171–7.
17. Geaghan S. Diagnostic laboratory technologies for the fetus and neonate with isoimmunization. Semin Perinatol. 2011;35(3):148–54.
18. Maisels M, Bhutani V, Bogen D, et al. Hyperbilirubinemia in the newborn infant > or = 35 weeks' gestation: an update with clarifications. Pediatrics. 2009;124(4):1193–8.
19. Rath M, Smits-Wintjens V, Lindenburg I, et al. Exchange transfusions and top-up transfusions in neonates with Kell haemolytic disease compared to Rh D haemolytic disease. Vox Sang. 2011;100(3):312–6.
20. Thayyil S, Milligan D. Single versus double volume exchange transfusion in jaundiced newborn infants. Cochrane Database Syst Rev. 2006;18(4):CD004592.
21. Gharehbaghi M, Hosseinpour S. Exchange transfusion in neonatal hyperbilirubinaemia: a comparison between citrated whole blood and reconstituted blood. Singapore Med J. 2010;51(8):641–4.

Chapter 5
Intrauterine Transfusions

Nahla Khalek

Indications

Red cell alloimmunization
Parvovirus B19 infection
Fetomaternal hemorrhage
Twin anemia polycythemia sequence
Placental and fetal tumors

Diagnosis

Intravascular Technique for Fetal Blood Sampling (FBS) and Intrauterine Transfusion (IUT)

Ultrasound-guided FBS can also be referred to as cordocentesis or percutaneous blood sampling (PUBS) and currently is the only procedure that provides direct access to the fetal circulation. This technique was first described in the 1980s [1, 2] and rapidly evolved from a fetoscopically guided procedure [3] to an ultrasound-guided procedure [2]. Suspected severe fetal anemia is now the most common clinical indication for FBS and IUT in the United States. The direct measurement of fetal hemoglobin and hematocrit to confirm clinically suspected fetal anemia can only be made by FBS. Currently there are numerous approaches to accomplish

N. Khalek, MD
Center for Fetal Diagnosis and Treatment, The Children's Hospital of Philadelphia, Perelman School of Medicine University of Pennsylvania, 34th Street and Civic Center Boulevard, Wood Building, 5th floor, Philadelphia, PA, USA
e-mail: khalekn@email.chop.edu

© Springer International Publishing Switzerland 2017
D.A. Sesok-Pizzini (ed.), *Neonatal Transfusion Practices*,
DOI 10.1007/978-3-319-42764-5_5

ultrasound-guided needle access to the fetal circulation: directly into the umbilical cord, either at the placental cord insertion (PCI), abdominal cord insertion (ACI), or into a free loop; into the intrahepatic vein (IHV); or, rarely, directly into the fetal heart via cardiocentesis. The use of maternal sedation is variable among centers, and many no longer administer intravenous sedation. Local anesthetic on the maternal skin at the site of needle insertion is often utilized by a majority of centers performing FBS/IUT [9–12]. The use of fetal paralytic agents was first reported in 1988 to reduce fetal movement during IUT [13]. Multiple centers performing IUT do use paralytic agents such as pancuronium, atracurium, or vecuronium. Pancuronium is long acting, whereas both atracurium and vecuronium are short acting. Paralytic agents may be useful and considered when larger transfusion volumes and longer operating times are anticipated or when fetal movements preclude maintaining safe vascular access [14–16]. Typically they are not used for diagnostic FBS or when the placenta is anterior and the PCI is readily accessible. An aseptic technique is utilized including a preprocedural antibacterial skin preparation to reduce the risk of infection. The insertion of the 20- or 22-gauge spinal needle is typically performed under direct ultrasound guidance, typically via ultrasound-guided freehand technique. The operator can self-guide, i.e., control the ultrasound transducer with one hand and the needle with the other, or an assistant can perform ultrasound guidance for needle insertion. With either approach, the operator follows the tip of the needle under continuous ultrasound guidance from percutaneous entry point to placement into the fetal circulation. When the umbilical cord is the target, typically it is the umbilical vein that is accessed as the umbilical arteries may vasoconstrict when punctured, leading to vasospasm and fetal bradycardia which may prompt an emergent delivery or fetal loss, based on gestational age at the time of the procedure. Choosing which gauge needle to use is dependent upon a number of factors including but not limited to indication for procedure (diagnostic vs. therapeutic), gestational age, maternal body habitus, and distance from skin to targeted vessel. There are distinct advantages of sampling and transfusing through the PCI that include the relative stability of the cord and shorter procedure times [9]. One important, potential, disadvantage to consider is the possibility of maternal cell contamination and needing to confirm that the sample obtained is completely fetal in origin. This is addressed by aspirating blood into a previously heparinized 1 cc syringe and submitting the sample to determine if the blood is fetal in origin via measuring mean corpuscular volume (MCV) or the Kleihauer-Betke test [10, 12, 17]. Traversing or penetrating the placenta in order to access a free loop or IHV raises concerns for the potential increased risk for fetomaternal hemorrhage and subsequently increased fetal death rates. A contemporary analysis of 615 cases of penetrating the placenta compared to 1560 cases of not penetrating the placenta [18] demonstrated no differences in duration of procedure, success rates, or fetal bradycardia. However, significant placental bleeding was associated in up to one third of cases with placental penetration and in no cases without placental penetration. There were also higher rates of fetal loss (3.6% vs. 1.3%, $P = 0.1$), umbilical cord bleeding (32% vs. 28.4%, $P < .05$), and lower gestational age at delivery.

Fetal Blood Specimen

When invasive testing is planned for suspected severe fetal anemia or thrombocytopenia, FBS is the procedure of choice, with availability of immediate transfusion if confirmed. The overall success rate of FBS is high, and blood samples can be obtained in >98 % of patients [4]. FBS should only be performed by experienced operators at centers with expertise in invasive fetal procedures when feasible.

Selection of RBCs

Donor units that are selected for IUT undergo the same screening and testing that occurs for any red cell donor unit, in addition to specific testing and RBC preparation. For IUTs, type O, Rh (D) negative blood is the most common type that is prepared for transfusion. In specific cases, blood negative to other antigens, such as when transfusing for Kell specific alloimmunization, may be required. All units are screened to confirm that they are CMV negative and they are also irradiated to minimize the risk of graft versus host reaction. Leukodepletion is also utilized. It is imperative that tightly packed donor cells yielding a hematocrit of 75–85 % are used so as to minimize the total volume transfused to the anemic fetus.

Volume Calculations

When it is determined that the fetus is a candidate for IUT, there are a variety of methods to determine the volume of blood to be transfused. Formulas are developed for determining the optimal transfusion volume factor in hematocrit of the donor unit, estimated fetal weight, and goal final hematocrit, all of which are determined prior to the IUT procedure. Factors that can modify the volume transfused at the time of the procedure include the presence of fetal hydrops and the fetal hematocrit at the time of initial sampling. In general, the final target fetal hematocrit should be aimed at 40–50 %. In fetuses over 24 weeks of gestation, one method for calculating the volume of donor blood for transfusion utilizes a coefficient multiplied by the estimated fetal weight to increase the fetal hematocrit by specific increments (see Table 5.1) [19, 20]. The formula assumes the hematocrit of the donor blood to be approximately 75 %:

$$\text{Estimated fetal weight (grams)} \times \text{coefficient} = \text{volume to transfuse}$$

There is also a web-based calculator that is freely available on www.perinatology. com that offers a standardized protocol for IUT [21].

Table 5.1 Method for calculating volume for fetal transfusion utilizing the transfusion coefficient [19]

Desired increment in Hct (%)	Transfusion coefficient
10	0.02
15	0.03
20	0.04
25	0.05
30	0.06

As ultrasound screening protocols for fetal anemia improve secondary to the increasing availability of assessing MCA Doppler PSV, anemic fetuses identified at 18–24 weeks are known to be at increased risk for complications secondary to IUT. In this population, the posttransfusion hematocrit threshold is lowered to 25 % or a fourfold increase from the pretransfusion value [22]. If it is clinically appropriate, a second transfusion may be performed within 48 h in an effort to raise the fetal hematocrit toward normal range for gestational age.

Complications

The most serious complication remains fetal distress intraoperatively or post-procedure. This may result in emergent cesarean delivery if gestational age appropriate, with the concomitant risks associated with prematurity, or fetal/neonatal demise. Fetal distress can occur secondary to cord rupture, spasm, tamponade from a cord hematoma, or excessive bleeding from the puncture site. In addition, volume overload, chorioamnionitis, preterm premature rupture of membranes, chorion-amnion separation, or preterm labor can contribute to fetal distress. Demise that occurs post-operatively can be explained by an already compromised fetal state or due to the procedure itself. Procedure-related fetal loss ranges from 0.9 to 4.9 % per procedure.

Counseling for FBS and IUT must include discussion about potential risks that may include but may not be limited to bleeding from puncture site (20–30 %), fetal bradycardia (5–10 %), pregnancy loss (≥1.3 %, depending on indication, gestational age, and placental penetration), and vertical transmission of hepatitis or human immunodeficiency virus, although there is currently insufficient published data to estimate this risk [4]. Based on small series examining vertical transmission with amniocentesis in these specific populations, the risks of vertical transmission appear to be very low and related to maternal viral load [5–8]).

Long-Term Neurodevelopmental Outcome After IUT

Based on over three decades of clinical data, the long-term neurodevelopmental outcome of children born after intrauterine transfusion (IUT) is generally considered to be favorable (see Table 5.2). The majority of data published relates to IUT for fetal

Table 5.2 Long-term neurodevelopmental outcomes in children treated with IUT for red cell alloimmunization

Author, year	Outcome measure	Cerebral palsy	NDI	Methodologic comments
Doyle et al. (1993) [24]	Bayley Scales	2.6 % (1/38)	7.9 % (3/38)	Controls not contemporaneous
Stewart et al. (1994) [25]	Cattell test	None (0/8)	None (0/8)	Insufficient power
Janssens et al. (1997) [26]	Van Weighenm POPS, Gesell schedules, Denver screening test	4 % (3/69)	10.1 % (7/69)	Wide age range of children
Hudon et al. (1998) [27]	Gesell schedules, McCarthy Scales	4.5 % (1/22)	NA	No controls High loss to follow-up rate
Grab et al. (1999) [28]	School performance	None (0/35)	NA	No controls No neurodevelopmental assessments
Farrant et al. (2001) [29]	Neurodevelopmental questionnaires	3.3 % (1/30)	NA	No controls No neurodevelopmental assessments
Harper et al. (2006) [30]	Differential Ability Scales, Wide Range Assessment, Gordon Diagnostic System	6.2 % (1/16)	12.5 % (2/16)	Insufficient power
Weisz et al. (2009) [31]	Neurodevelopmental questionnaire	None (0/40)	NA	No controls No neurodevelopmental tests
Lindenberg (2011)	Touwen, Bayley Scales, Wechsler Scales	2.1 % (6/291)	4.8 % (14/291)	No controls

Table adapted from Van Klink et al. [33]
NDI neurodevelopmental impairment defined as CP, cognitive functioning or developmental delay, blindness, or deafness. *NA* data not available

anemia secondary to red cell alloimmunization. Long-term neurodevelopmental outcomes in children who received IUT as secondary to parvovirus B19 infection and fetomaternal hemorrhage are less well established when compared to outcomes in children who received IUT for red cell alloimmunization. Based on case series reported, there is a suggestion that the incidence of severe neurodevelopmental delay and cerebral palsy is higher when compared to standardized population controls, which may reflect the association between intrauterine fetal infection and fetal cerebral injury [23]. Limitations to long-term follow-up that have been identified include small sample size, paucity of controls, ambiguous criteria for what constitutes major neurodevelopmental impairment, and the lack of regular application of standardized neurodevelopmental assessments [33]. The strongest predictor for adverse neurodevelopmental outcomes was the prenatal diagnosis of hydrops. Other factors include the number of IUTs performed, premature delivery, and concomitant neonatal morbidity as well as parental socioeconomic status [32, 33].

An improved understanding of the effect of IUT and fetal anemia on child development longitudinally will allow for more accurate prenatal counseling, and targeted interventions aimed at optimizing these long-term outcomes.

References

Intravascular Techniques for FBS

1. Bang J, Bock JE, Trolle D. Ultrasound guided fetal intravenous transfusion for severe rhesus hemolytic disease. Br Med J. 1982;284:373–4.
2. Daffos F, Capella-Pavlovsky M, Forestier F. A new procedure for fetal blood sampling in utero: preliminary results of fifty-three cases. Am J Obstet Gynecol. 1983;146:985–7.
3. Rodeck CH, Campbell S. Umbilical cord insertion as a source of pure fetal blood for prenatal diagnosis. Lancet. 1979;1:1244–5.
4. Berry SM, Stone J, Norton ME, Johnson D, Berghella V. Fetal blood sampling. Am J Obstet Gynecol. 2013;209(3):170–80.
5. Alexander JM, Ramus R, Jackson G, Sercely B, Wendel GD. Risk of hepatitis B transmission after amniocentesis in chronic hepatitis B carriers. Infect Dis Obstet Gynecol. 1999;7:283–6.
6. Delamare C, Carbonne B, Heim N, et al. Detection of hepatitis C virus RNA (HCV RNA) in amniotic fluid: a prospective study. J Hepatol. 1999;31:416–20.
7. Somigliana E, Bucceri AM, Tibaldi C, et al. Early invasive diagnostic techniques in pregnant women who are infected with the HIV: a multicenter case series. Am J Obstet Gynecol. 2005;193:437–42.
8. Towers CV, Asrat T, Rumney P. The presence of hepatitis B surface antigen and deoxyribonucleic acid in amniotic fluid and cord blood. Am J Obstet Gynecol. 2001;184:1514–20.
9. Tangshewinsirikul C, Wanapirak C, Piyamongkol W, Sirichotiyakul S, Tongsong T. Effect of cord puncture site in cordocentesis at mid-pregnancy on pregnancy outcomes. Prenat Diagn. 2001;31:861–64.
10. Tongsong T, Wanapirak C, Kunavikatikul C, Sirirchotiyakul S, Piyamongkol W, Chanprapaph P. Cordocentesis at 16–24 weeks of gestation: experience of 1,320 cases. Prenat Diagn. 2000;20:224.
11. Aina-Mumuney AJ, Holcroft CJ, Blakemore KJ, et al. Intrahepatic vein for fetal blood sampling: one center's experience. Am J Obstet Gynecol. 2008;198:387.e1–e6.
12. Boulout P, Deschamps F, Lefort G, et al. Pure fetal blood samples obtained by cordocentesis: technical aspects of 322 cases. Prenat Diagn. 1990;10:93–100.
13. Copel JA, Grannum PA, Harrison D, Hobbins JC. The use of intravenous pancuronium bromide to produce fetal paralysis during intravascular transfusion. Am J Obstet Gynecol. 1988;158:170–1.
14. Moise KJ, Deter RL, Kirshon B, Adam K, Patton DE, Carpenter RJ. Intravenous pancuronium bromide for fetal neuromuscular blockade during intrauterine transfusion for red-cell alloimmunization. Obstet Gynecol. 1989;74:905–8.
15. Bernstein HH, Chitkara U, Plosker H, Gettes M, Berkowitz RL. Use of atracurium besylate to arrest fetal activity during intrauterine intravascular transfusions. Obstet Gynecol. 1988;72:813–16.
16. Leveque C, Murat I, Toubas F, Poissonnier MH, Brossard Y, Saint-Maurice C. Fetal neuromuscular blockade with vecuronium bromide: studies during intravascular intrauterine transfusion in isoimmunized pregnancies. Anesthesiology. 1992;76:642–44.
17. Liao C, Wei J, Li Q, Li L, Li J, Li D. Efficacy and safety of cordocentesis for prenatal diagnosis. Int Gyencol Obstet. 2006;93:13–7.
18. Boupaijit K, Wanapirak C, Piyamongkol W, Sirichotiyakul S, Tongsong T. Effect of placenta penetration during cordocentesis at mid pregnancy on fetal outcomes. Prenat Diagn. 2012;32:83–7.

Volume Calculations

19. Mari G, Norton ME, Stone J, Berghella V, Sciscione AC, Tate D, Schenone MH. Society for Maternal-Fetal Medicine (SMFM) Clinical Guideline #8: the fetus at risk for anemia-diagnosis and management. Am J Obstet Gynecol. 2015;212(6):697–710.
20. Moise KJ, Whitecar PW. Antenatal therapy for hemolytic disease. In: Hadley A, Soothill P, editors. Alloimmune disorders of pregnancy. Anemia, thrombocytopenia and neutropenia in the fetus and newborn. Cambridge, UK: Cambridge University Press; 2002.
21. http://perinatology.com/protocols/rhc.htm.
22. Radunovic N, Lockwood CJ, Alvarez M, Plecas D, Chitkara U, Berkowitz RL. The severely anemic and hydropic isoimmune fetus: changes in fetal hematocrit associated with intrauterine death. Obstet Gynecol. 1992;79:390–93.

Complications: ND Outcomes

23. DeJong EP, Lindenberg IT, van Klink JM, Oepkes D, van Kamp IL, Wlather FJ, Lopriore E. Intrauterine transfusion for parvovirus B19 infection: long term neurodevelopmental outcome. Am J Obstet Gynecol. 2012;206:e1–5.
24. Doyle LW, Kelly EA, Rickards AL, Ford GW, Callanan C. Sensorineural outcome at two years for survivors of erythroblastosis treated with fetal intravascular transfusions. Obstet Gynecol. 1993;81:931–5.
25. Stewart G, Day RE, Del PC, Whittle MJ, Turner TL, Holland BM. Developmental outcome after intravascular intrauterine transfusion for rhesus hemolytic disease. Arch Dis Child Fetal Neonatal Ed. 1994;70:F52–3.
26. Janssens HM, de Haan MJ, van Kemp IL, Brand R, Kanhai HH, Veen S. Outcome for children treated with fetal intravascular transfusions because of severe blood group antagonism. J Pediatr. 1997;131:373–80.
27. Hudon L, Moise KJ, Hegemier SE, Hill RM, Moise AA, Smith EO, et al. Long term neurodevelopmental outcome after intrauterine transfusion for the treatment of fetal hemolytic disease. Am J Obstet Gynecol. 1998;81:931–35.
28. Grab D, Paulus WE, Bommer A, Bucjk G, Terinde R. Treatment of fetal erythroblastosis by intravascular transfusions: outcomes at 6 years. Obstet Gynecol. 1999;93:165–8.
29. Farrant B, Battin M, Roberts A. Outcomes of infants receiving in utero transfusions for hemolytic disease. N Z Med J. 2001;114:400–3.
30. Harper DC, Swigle HM, Weiner CP, Bonthius DJ, Aylward GP, Widness JA. Long term neurodevelopmental outcome and brain volume after treatment for hydrops fetalis by in utero intravascular transfusion. Am J Obstet Gynecol. 2006;195:192–200.
31. Weisz B, Rosenbaum O, Chayen B, Peltz R, Feldman B, Lipitz S. Outcome of severely anemic fetuses treated by intrauterine transfusions. Arch Dis Child Fetal Neonatal Ed. 2009;94:F201–4.
32. Lindenberg ITM, Smits-Wintjens VE, Van Klink JMM, Verduin E, Van Kamp IL, Walther FJ, et al. Long term neurodevelopmental outcome after intrauterine transfusion for hemolytic disease of the fetus/newborn: the LOTUS study. Am J Obstet Gynecol. 2012;206:141.e1–8.
33. Van Klink JMM, Koopman HM, Oepkes D, Walther FJ, Lopriore E. Long term neurodevelopmental outcome after intrauterine transfusion for fetal anemia. Early Hum Dev. 2011;87:589–93.

Chapter 6
Adverse Reactions

Jamie E. Kallan and Kelley E. Capocelli

Abbreviations

2,3-DPG	2,3-Diphosphoglycerate
AHTRs	Acute hemolytic transfusion reactions
ARDs	Acute respiratory distress syndrome
BRMs	Biologic response modifiers
CMV	*Cytomegalovirus*
DIC	Disseminated intravascular coagulation
ECMO	Extracorporeal membrane oxygenation
ESAs	Erythropoiesis-stimulating agents
FNHTRs	Febrile nonhemolytic transfusion reactions
G6PD	Glucose-6-phosphate dehydrogenase
HLA	Human leukocyte antigens
HNAs	Human neutrophil antigens
HTRs	Hemolytic transfusion reactions
IgG	Immunoglobulin G
NEC	Necrotizing enterocolitis
NICU	Neonatal intensive care unit
RBCs	Red blood cells
TACO	Transfusion-associated circulatory overload
TA-GVHD	Transfusion-associated graft-versus-host disease
TANEC	Transfusion-associated necrotizing enterocolitis
TRALI	Transfusion-related acute lung injury

J.E. Kallan, MD (✉)
Department of Pathology, University of Colorado Hospital, Aurora, CO, USA
e-mail: Jamie.Kallan@UCDenver.edu

K.E. Capocelli, MD
Pathology and Laboratory Medicine, Children's Hospital Colorado, Aurora, CO, USA
e-mail: kelley.capocelli@childrenscolorado.org

© Springer International Publishing Switzerland 2017
D.A. Sesok-Pizzini (ed.), *Neonatal Transfusion Practices*,
DOI 10.1007/978-3-319-42764-5_6

Red Cell Storage Lesions and Metabolic Imbalances

When red blood cells are stored, they undergo a variety of physiologic changes known as red cell storage lesions. Changes associated with red cell storage lesions include increased extracellular potassium, decreased 2,3-diphophoglycerate (2,3-DPG), and increased plasma hemoglobin. These lesions are accelerated with irradiation. While not considered to be true transfusion reactions, red cell storage lesions can cause harmful side effects to neonatal patients undergoing transfusions. Given their small blood volumes, neonates are at an increased risk of developing metabolic imbalances following transfusion secondary to red cell storage lesions. This is due, in part, to the inability of their immature liver to effectively metabolize citrate and the reduced glomerular filtration rate associated with kidney immaturity that causes slower excretion of excess potassium, acid, and calcium. Hypocalcemia may occur after rapid transfusion of citrate, and alkalosis may develop after metabolism of large amounts of citrate. Because of this, infants less than 4 months of age may develop hyperkalemia, acid–base imbalances, or hypocalcemia following large-volume transfusions. In addition, the preservative solutions used to increase the shelf life of blood products can contain solutes causing diuresis, altered blood volume, and potentially altered cerebral blood flow leading to increased risk of intraventricular hemorrhage [40, 46].

Hyperkalemia

The increase in storage-related extracellular potassium along with the impaired renal function in neonates due to disease or prematurity can put them at increased risk for transfusion-associated hyperkalemia. This occurs primarily during large-volume rapid transfusions such as occur with extracorporeal membrane oxygenation (ECMO), exchange transfusions, or during surgery. Small-volume transfusions administered at a slow rate have been shown to have little effect on serum potassium concentrations on neonates.

For example, a typical unit of red blood cells (RBCs) contains a starting extracellular potassium concentration of 5–10 mEq/L. Sometimes due to donor issues, the unit may start out with higher levels of potassium. During refrigerated storage, the intracellular potassium within RBCs continues to be released into the extracellular space due to reduction in the activity of the Na–K ATPase pump. The type of anticoagulant-preservative solution used in the storage of RBCs influences the amount of potassium leak. For example, after 35 days, the concentration of extracellular potassium within a unit of red blood cells preserved with CPDA-1 can reach 70–80 mEq/L. In contrast, after 42 days the concentration of extracellular potassium within a unit of red blood cells preserved with AS-1, AS-3, or AS-5 reaches approximately half of that amount at 40–50 mEq/L. Increases in extracellular potassium secondary to hemolysis can also occur due to excessive heating or freezing of the unit, the use of hypo-osmotic solutions during RBC transfusion, bacterial contamination, mechanical hemolysis from transfusion through small-gauge needles, and exposure to UV light in patients undergoing phototherapy.

Life-threatening effects of hyperkalemia, especially when administered through a central or intracardiac line where high concentrations of potassium are being rapidly delivered to the heart without first being filtered through the kidneys, include cardiac arrest and death. In order to reduce the risk of hyperkalemia in neonatal patients, transfusion with fresh RBCs is recommended. Washing a red cell unit can also be an effective means of removing extracellular potassium, especially for units that have been stored for >24 h or have been irradiated >24 h before transfusion as irradiation potentiates potassium release. However, this effect is only temporary with extracellular potassium rising again following washing (up to 5 mEq/L in non-irradiated and 12 mEq/L in irradiated units after 24 h).

Irradiation of blood products accelerates the rate of red cell storage lesions, especially the extracellular leakage of potassium >12 h after irradiation. Therefore, it is recommended that red blood cells be irradiated as close to the time of transfusion as possible, especially for large-volume transfusions (>20 mL/kg) in order to minimize the accumulation of extracellular potassium. In neonates receiving aliquots, it is preferable to irradiate only the aliquot being transfused instead of the entire parent unit. This is only possible if a hospital has an irradiator on site, which is preferable for institutions who routinely administer large-volume transfusions to neonatal patients. If hospitals do not have an irradiator and must receive irradiated blood from an outside source, hyperkalemia may be a concern if the irradiated unit is not transfused immediately (within 12 h of irradiation). There have been case reports and anecdotal reports of infant deaths caused by infusions of high concentrations of extracellular potassium in as little as 24 h after irradiation [23]. If the unit cannot be used in a neonatal patient within 12 h of irradiation, then the irradiated unit should be assigned to a larger child or adult patient instead.

Because of these time constraints, communication between the clinical team and the blood bank is essential to coordinate the time of transfusion in order to help reduce the risk of hyperkalemia. Ideally, procedures should be in place to rapidly irradiate and dispense such units. If irradiation cannot be performed fast enough for the patient's transfusion needs, policies should be in place to evaluate the risk of transfusion-associated hyperkalemia, transfusion-associated graft-versus-host disease, and transfusion delays. Alternatively, if a neonate requires large-volume transfusion, it may be helpful for the transfusing provider to preemptively treat the infant for hyperkalemia. Calcium boluses can be given up front. In some instances, albumin or glucose could also be utilized.

2,3-Diphosphoglycerate

2,3-DPG is a molecule that is essential for red blood cell metabolism. It normally works to shift the hemoglobin–oxygen dissociation curve to the right, increasing the ability of red blood cells to release oxygen into tissue. During storage, the amount of 2,3-DPG diminishes rapidly which shifts the hemoglobin–oxygen dissociation curve to the left, thereby reducing the ability of red blood cells to release oxygen into tissue. By storage day 21, the amount of 2,3-DPG is completely depleted from the red blood cell unit. Studies in adults have shown that it takes between 3 and 8 h for 2,3-DPG to be regenerated after one unit of RBCs has been transfused and that older patients are able to compensate for the resulting hypoxia by increasing their heart rate. However, infants younger than 4 months old are not able to compensate as effectively. In addition, sick neonates with respiratory distress syndrome or sepsis may have even lower levels of intracellular 2,3-DPG. Because of this, it has been suggested that fresh blood products be used for neonates undergoing large-volume transfusions in order to increase the amount of 2,3-DPG that they receive. As with hyperkalemia, the need for fresh blood products in small-volume transfusions is unnecessary as the decreased amount of 2,3-DPG is unlikely to reduce the amount of oxygen available to tissues.

Special Processing of Blood Components

Neonates comprise a special patient population that requires additional manipulation of blood products (i.e., washing, irradiation, bedside filtration, or concentration) which can extend the preparation time, shorten the shelf life, and alter the composition of the blood product (i.e., hyperkalemia) being transfused. This special processing of blood products is primarily performed in order to reduce the risk of the infant's immature immune system from exposure to many infectious and noninfectious complications of transfusion. Much of an infant's humoral (antibody-mediated) immunity is provided by the mother through the placental transfer of immunoglobulins in utero, which consist predominantly of the immunoglobulin G (IgG) class of molecules. After delivery, the mother is no longer able to provide these antibodies to the infant for immune protection. In addition, an infant's cellular immunity is incompletely developed at birth, making them especially susceptible to transfusion-associated graft-versus-host disease.

Irradiation

The irradiation of blood is performed on cellular products in order to prevent transfusion-associated graft-versus-host disease (TA-GVHD). It is recommended that cellular blood products be irradiated for the following patients: premature infants weighing <1200 g at birth, any patient with a known or suspected cellular immune deficiency, any patient with significant immunosuppression related to chemotherapy or radiation treatment, and any patient receiving HLA-matched or crossmatched platelet components. In addition, parents or other blood relatives who wish to be a direct blood donor for an infant must have the donated units irradiated. For practical purposes, many institutions choose to set an age in which all neonates under the set age will receive irradiated blood. The irradiation of blood products may generate increased operational costs, time delays, and damage to red blood cells.

Washing

The washing of RBCs is most commonly performed in order to remove excess extracellular potassium or preservative solutions in large-volume transfusions. This process also reduces the number of leukocytes, although not enough to label the washed product as leukocyte reduced. Unfortunately, when a unit of RBCs is washed, up to 20% of the red cell mass can be lost. In addition, because washing usually occurs in an open system, the expiration date of washed RBCs decreases to 24 h. The reduction in shelf life of washed products is in part due to the increased possibility of external contamination or other technical errors, and also because the preservative solution has been removed, thereby affecting the viability of the red blood cells. Because the amount of potassium and adenine in aliquot transfusions of <20 mL/kg have not been shown to be detrimental, the benefits of washing the blood product in small-volume transfusions must be weighed against the potential risks. In many cases, washing is unnecessary and may inadvertently expose the patient to increased risk. If, however, the patient requires a large-volume transfusion, the transfusion is being administered through a central or intracardiac line, the blood product is greater than 7–14 days old, or the blood product has been irradiated >12 h before the transfusion, then washing could be considered in order to reduce the amount of extracellular potassium. In addition, it is strongly encouraged that any RBCs or platelets which were donated by the mother be washed in order to remove maternal plasma and reduce the risk of hemolytic disease of the fetus and newborn, neonatal alloimmune cytopenia, and transfusion-related acute lung injury (TRALI).

In neonates, the most common indication for washing platelets is to remove ABO-incompatible antibodies. For example, infants with neonatal alloimmune thrombocytopenia must receive transfusions from a donor who lacks the particular antigen, which is often the mother. However, the donors who lack the antigen will have the corresponding antibody to that antigen. Because of this, it is necessary to wash the donor platelets prior to transfusion in order to remove the offending antibody. Platelets should also be washed prior to being transfused in patients with severe allergic transfusion reactions, IgA deficiency, and anti-IgA antibodies. However, the washing of platelets can result in a loss of up to 50–75% of platelets with an associated loss in activation and function. One study has suggested that washing platelets with ACD-A buffered saline helps retain platelet function when compared to washing platelets with saline [53, 61]. In addition, washing platelets with an automated method via cell processor may provide a loss of only 8% of platelets with more consistent results. Washing platelets reduces the shelf life to 4 h. If, as often occurs in the neonatal population, the volume of washed platelets exceeds the transfusion need, the remaining unused washed platelets will be wasted.

Leukocyte Reduction

The risk of acquiring *Cytomegalovirus* (CMV) by transfusion is between 1 and 3 %. Signs and symptoms of CMV infection in neonates are highly variable and can range from asymptomatic seroconversion to death. At high risk of transfusion-transmitted CMV infection are low-birth-weight infants (<1200 g) who are born to seronegative mothers. Because of this, it is recommended that low-birth-weight infants who are born to seronegative mothers receive CMV-reduced-risk blood. While deglycerolized, washed RBCs and blood from seronegative donors have been shown to reduce the risk of transfusion-transmitted CMV infection; the most common approach utilized today to reduce the risk of CMV transmission is leukocyte reduction.

Photochemical Pathogen Inactivation Treatment

A photochemical treatment process has been developed and approved for use in Europe since 2002 and has been shown to inactivate viruses, bacteria, protozoa, and leukocytes that may contaminate blood products. This technique uses amotosalen, a synthetic psoralen that penetrates cellular and nuclear membranes and covalently crosslinks to the nucleic acid–base pairs upon exposure to low-energy UVA light to block DNA and RNA replication [74]. This process renders leukocytes and pathogens unable to cause disease while maintaining the function of the plasma or platelet components, which do not require nucleic acid replication for therapeutic effect. Extensive preclinical safety programs demonstrated the absence of any relevant toxic effects in juvenile or adult animals. No amotosalen-related effects on clinical signs, body weight, hematology, clinical chemistry, urinalysis, gross pathology, or histopathology were noted despite administration of amotosalen concentrations as high as 48 times the standard exposure in adult patients [8]. An active hemovigilance program was implemented in order to prospectively examine adverse events associated with the transfusion of photochemically treated platelets [50, 51]. A prospective study over 7 years examined 4067 patients who received 19,175 platelet transfusions containing the photochemical treatment process and found a similar safety profile as conventional platelet components [50, 51] with a lower rate of acute transfusion reactions (9.5 % of patients transfused with platelets in plasma plus photochemical additive solution vs. 15.5 % of patients transfused with conventional platelets suspended in plasma). No cases of TRALI, TA-GVHD, transfusion-transmitted infection, or death were attributed to the transfusion of photochemical treatment-processed platelets [34].

Transmission of Infectious Disease

Despite improvements in donor screening and testing of blood components, every transfusion is associated with a risk of infectious disease transmission. For example, current testing is unreliable during the window period between donor infections and seroconversion. In addition, the risk of transfusion-transmitted infectious diseases increases with exposure. Given their small size, neonates are often transfused with small-volume aliquots, which are often collected from the original unit of blood via an opened port system. When an open collection system is used, the primary unit of blood expires 24 h after the initial aliquot is produced. Any subsequent transfusion requirements occurring after 24 h require an aliquot to be produced from a new primary unit. Because of this, over the course of a hospital stay, a neonatal patient could be exposed to multiple donors, thereby putting them at increased risk for disease transmission or other transfusion-related complications. On average, premature infants weighing <1 kg are exposed to more than five donors during a single hospital stay if an opened port system is utilized for aliquot production. When a sterile collecting device is used, blood products are able to be stored for longer periods of time, and the neonate is able to receive multiple aliquots from the same primary unit. This decreases their exposure to multiple blood donors and the associated complications. In addition, this minimizes the wastage of blood components. However, sometimes there may be concern for continually exposing a patient to the same donor. For example, if the dedicated donor blood contains a previously undetected infectious disease or a harmful substance, this can introduce an increased dose of a life-threatening or toxic substance.

Several measures have been adopted in order to prevent or eliminate the potential infectious risk from the transfusion of blood products including solvent/detergents used in viral reduction of pooled plasma and methylene blue used in single-donor plasma. While these methods are very effective in eliminating lipid-enveloped viruses, they have little to no effect on nonenveloped pathogens. These methods are also not licensed for use in the United States. As previously mentioned, new photochemical pathogen inactivation treatments have been shown to be effective at inactivating bacteria, viruses, protozoa, and donor leukocyte contaminants within plasma and platelet units while preserving to therapeutic effectiveness of the blood component. While potential hazards of introducing amotosalen and UVA light (the components used in photochemical pathogen inactivation treatments) include genotoxicity, carcinogenicity, and phototoxicity, no specific target organ toxicity, phototoxicity, or reproductive toxicity has been observed [9, 10].

The use of recombinant human erythropoietin has been shown to reduce donor exposures in neonatal patients while minimizing the severity of their anemia. Erythropoietin stimulates the bone marrow to produce red blood cells with relatively small side effects, therefore reducing transfusion requirements. Studies evaluating the non-hematopoietic effects of erythropoiesis-stimulating agents (ESAs) have suggested that they may also be neuroprotective by promoting oligodendrogenesis, decreasing inflammation, decreasing oxidative injury, and decreasing apoptosis. One study found that the weekly administration of ESAs in preterm infants resulted in higher cognitive and object permanence scores with a lower incidence of cerebral palsy at 18–22 months corrected age [48]. Therefore, ESAs may not only be a beneficial therapy in preterm infants at risk for anemia but may also act as a neuroprotective agent which can improve neurodevelopmental outcomes.

Sepsis

Bacterial infections are more frequently associated with the transfusion of platelets than any other blood product. Despite extensive donor screening and testing, transfusion-transmitted infections continue to occur. Fever, chills, and hypotension are the most common symptoms of sepsis that occur during or shortly after the transfusion. These symptoms may overlap with other transfusion-associated reactions, including acute hemolytic transfusion reactions (AHTR) or febrile nonhemolytic transfusion reactions (FNHTRs). In cases of suspected posttransfusion sepsis, visual examination of the returned blood component should be conducted in order to detect changes in color along with any bubbles or frothiness. In addition, a Gram stain should be performed on the returned blood component along with cultures of both the returned blood component and a posttransfusion blood sample from the patient. The key to diagnosing transfusion-associated sepsis is to culture the same organism from both the patient and the remainder of the blood component. Any intravenous solutions that were administered concomitantly should be cultured as well. Supportive measures including broad-spectrum antibiotics may be started to help treat the patient.

Febrile Nonhemolytic Transfusion Reactions

A febrile nonhemolytic transfusion reaction (FNHTR) is defined as a greater than 1 C increase in temperature above 37 C which is associated with transfusion and for which no other cause of fever is identifiable. It is important to note that a preexisting fever may mask a FNHTR in febrile patients. FNHTRs are caused by leukocyte antibodies and/or accumulated cytokines within a cellular blood component. It is thought that the rise in temperature is a result of recipient HLA antibodies reacting with antigens present on transfused lymphocytes, granulocytes, or platelets that incite an antigen–antibody reaction and a release in cytokines.

Associated symptoms may include shaking, chills, increased respiratory rate, change in blood pressure, and feelings of anxiety. The onset of symptoms usually occurs while the blood product is being transfused but may occur up to 2 h after the transfusion has been completed. Although they may cause discomfort and changes in hemodynamics and respiration, FNHTRs are benign. However, it is important to distinguish symptoms of a FNHTR from those that may overlap with other more serious transfusion reactions such as hemolytic transfusion reactions (HTRs), sepsis, and TRALI. Other signs and symptoms along with laboratory data can be used to help determine which transfusion reaction occurred, with FNHTR being a diagnosis of exclusion.

When FNHTR is suspected, the transfusion should be stopped immediately and a transfusion reaction workup initiated. Antipyretics should be administered, and once symptoms subside, the patient may once again be safely transfused. In order to help prevent FNHTR, prestorage leukocyte reduction can be used in order to reduce the number of residual leukocytes to less than 5×10^6 in red blood cells and apheresis platelets. Antipyretics and leukocyte reduction have been shown to decrease the frequency of FNHTR without compromising the ability to detect serious transfusion complications.

Acute Hemolytic Transfusion Reactions

While a relatively uncommon complication of blood product transfusions (estimated to occur in 1 per 76,000 transfusions) [73], acute hemolytic transfusion reactions (AHTRs) occur due to the transfusion of ABO-incompatible blood products. Symptoms are a result of preformed antigens within the recipient that interact with donor antigens present in the blood component being transfused. The most severe AHTRs occur in red cell transfusions that are ABO incompatible with the recipient's isohemagglutinins. Preformed IgM or IgG antibodies recognize the corresponding donor red cell antigens leading to acute intravascular destruction of the transfused cells resulting in hemolysis, hemoglobinemia, and hemoglobinuria. IgM and, when present in high enough concentrations, IgG antibodies can activate complement leading to the production of C3a, C3b, and C5a which are anaphylatoxins that coat the donor red blood cells, assemble a membrane attack complex, and lead to intravascular hemolysis. C3a and C5a also promote the release of histamine and serotonin from mast cells resulting in vasodilation and smooth muscle contraction predominantly within the respiratory and gastrointestinal tracts. C3a and C5a also stimulate monocytes, macrophages, endothelial cells, and platelets to release cytokines, leukotrienes, free radicals, nitric oxide, interleukin-8 (IL-8), tumor necrosis factor alpha (TNFα), IL-1β, IL-6, and monocyte chemoattractant protein-1 into the bloodstream. The antigen–antibody complex itself stimulates the release of bradykinin and norepinephrine, and phagocytosis of IgG-coated red blood cells leads to additional cytokine release [16].

ABO-incompatible plasma found in apheresis platelets has also been shown to cause hemolysis of the recipient's red blood cells. This scenario typically occurs when group O platelets from donors with high anti-A antibody titers are transfused to group A patients [28, 60]. Unlike AHTRs associated with red blood cell transfusions, AHTRs associated with platelet transfusions tend to be less clinically significant. In the presence of non-ABO antibodies, complement activation does not proceed to completion, leading to extravascular hemolysis with red blood cells that are coated in C3b or IgG being rapidly removed from circulation by phagocytosis. Figure 6.1 is a compatibility chart for red blood cells, whole blood, and plasma products (platelets, plasma, and cryoprecipitate).

Blood type	Compatible red blood cells	Compatible whole blood	Compatible platelets and plasma
O positive	O+, O−	O+, O−	All types
O negative	O−	O−	All types
B positive	B+, B−, O+, O−	B+, B−	Any B or AB
B negative	B−,O−	B−	Any B or AB
A positive	A+, A−, O+, O−	A+, A−	Any B or AB
A negative	A−, O−	A−,	Any B or AB
AB positive	All types	AB+, AB−	Any AB
AB negative	All types	AB−	Any AB

Fig. 6.1 Compatibility chart for red blood cells, whole blood, and plasma products (platelets, plasma, and cryoprecipitate)

The most common symptoms associated with AHTRs include fever, chills, rigors, abdominal pain, chest pain, back pain, and flank pain. In severe cases, one can see hypotension, dyspnea, and dark urine due to intravascular hemolysis which can progress to shock or even disseminated intravascular coagulation (DIC) in some cases. In neonates, a relatively large amount of incompatible blood may have been transfused before acute hemolysis is recognized. However, as soon as an AHTR is suspected, immediate cessation of the transfusion is critical. The unit of blood being transfused should be returned to the blood bank for investigation and root-cause analysis. If a large amount of incompatible blood has been transfused, red cell exchange transfusions may be considered using antigen-negative blood.

Saline should be administered to the patient in order to help treat hypotension and to ensure adequate renal blood flow. Urine output should be closely monitored, with a goal urine flow rate of greater than 1 mL/kg/h. Low-dose dopamine hydrochloric acid may also be administered in order to provide an inotropic cardiac effect while selectively improving renal blood flow, and furosemide can further enhance renal cortical blood flow and urine output. If urine output remains low after infusion of 1 L of saline, this may indicate that acute tubular necrosis of the kidneys has occurred, and the patient may be at risk for developing pulmonary edema. A nephrologist should be consulted as oliguric renal failure may lead to hyperkalemia with subsequent cardiac arrest. The presence of metabolic acidosis and uremia may indicate the need for dialysis.

Disseminated intravascular coagulation (DIC) is another potentially life-threatening complication of AHTR. The antigen–antibody interaction may active the intrinsic pathway of the clotting cascade, resulting in the activation of Factor XII. This can result in hypotension, vascular permeability, and vasodilation. Activation of complement, interleukin-1, and tumor necrosis factor-α can increase the expression of tissue factor, which results in activation of the extrinsic pathway of the clotting cascade that is associated with the development of DIC. DIC characteristically results in microvascular thrombi formation, ischemic damage to tissue and organs, consumption of platelets, fibrinogen and coagulation factors, and activation of fibrinolysis [57]. Patients may experience symptoms ranging from generalized oozing to uncontrollable bleeding. Patients in DIC may require transfusion support with platelets, fresh frozen plasma, cryoprecipitate, and activated protein C. The use of heparin in treating DIC is controversial.

The severity of symptoms correlates with the amount of incompatible blood transfused. Therefore, prompt recognition and immediate cessation of the transfusion can help to prevent progression of AHTRs. Many of the signs and symptoms of AHTRs may overlap with other acute transfusion reactions. Fever, chills, and hypotension may also be seen in sepsis and TRALI. In addition, a patient's underlying condition may present with symptoms similar to an AHTR. For example, patients with glucose-6-phosphate dehydrogenase (G6PD) deficiency may experience hemolysis following a transfusion, and patients with autoimmune hemolytic anemia or sickle cell disease may experience fever and hypotension as a result of their condition. It is also important to differentiate between immune and nonimmune causes of hemolysis. For example, transfusion-associated hemolysis can occur as a result of the improper shipment conditions, inappropriate storage temperature, or incomplete deglycerolization of frozen red blood cells. As often occurs in the neonatal population, mechanical hemolysis can occur by using inappropriately small needle core sizes, employing rapid pressure infusers, the improper use of blood warmers, or the simultaneous transfusion of red blood cells with hypotonic solutions. Although these symptoms may not represent a true AHTR, it is always best to immediately stop a transfusion whenever a transfusion reaction is suspected as an AHTR can occur rapidly with the transfusion of as little as 10 mL of ABO-incompatible blood.

Prevention is crucial in AHTRs due to the fact that the most common cause is transfusing blood components to the wrong patient due to clerical and human errors. Identifying the wrong patient, patient sample, and blood unit have been cited as the most common causes of mistransfusion. Institutional policies and procedures should be in place to identify, correct, and minimize such errors. In addition, concentrating or volume reduction helps to minimize transfusion-incompatible plasma.

Transfusion-Associated Allergic Reactions

Transfusion-associated allergic reactions are common, occurring in approximately 1–3 % of all transfusions and accounting for 13–33 % of all transfusion reactions [17, 72]. Allergic reactions occur most commonly with the transfusion of plasma or platelets. Transfusion-associated allergic reactions can range from more common mild urticaria to less common life-threatening anaphylaxis. Urticaria, or hives, is a pruritic red, raised, and swollen wheals on the skin which can occur anywhere on the body and can vary in size. While urticaria can last hours to several days after the transfusion has been stopped, they tend to respond quickly to antihistamines. In more severe cases, urticaria may be associated with angioedema. Angioedema is an accumulation of fluid beneath the skin that commonly occurs around the eyes and lips. Angioedema occurring around the throat, tongue, or lungs can cause respiratory distress. A more serious complication is an anaphylactoid transfusion reaction, which can include urticaria and angioedema with additional cardiovascular symptoms including hypotension, tachycardia, arrhythmia, shock, loss of consciousness, or cardiac arrest. When the respiratory system is often involved, wheezing, stridor, and dyspnea can be seen. Approximately 30 % of these patients will also experience gastrointestinal symptoms such as nausea, vomiting, diarrhea, and abdominal cramps.

Transfusion-associated allergic reactions that are more severe and progress beyond urticaria may be seen in IgA-deficient patients and are caused by the reaction of anti-IgA antibodies in the recipient to IgA in the donated blood component. While IgA deficiency is estimated to occur in up to 1 in 700 people of European ancestry, only a small percentage of people go on to create antibodies to IgA. This may reflect the difference between patients with an absolute IgA deficiency and those with decreased but detectable amounts of IgA but form subclass-specific antibodies (i.e., anti-IgA1, anti-IgA2) depending on which component they are lacking. While it is important to recognize an IgA deficiency in patients receiving a blood transfusion, it is important to note that that the majority of anaphylactoid reactions are caused by allergens other than IgA [59]. Other known triggers of anaphylactoid reactions include antibodies against haptoglobin [63], penicillin, ethylene oxide, and C4 complement [37].

Transfusion-associated allergic reactions most commonly occur in response to allergens within the blood component being transfused and less commonly by antibodies from an allergic donor. Preformed IgE antibodies in the recipient interact with allergens present within the blood component, usually a plasma protein. Mast cells are activated by the binding of IgE on their surface to antigens in a type I hypersensitivity reaction [25]. This reaction causes degranulation of the mast cells including release of histamine, chemotactic factors, proteases, and proteoglycans. Secondary mediators such as cytokines, arachidonic acid metabolites, leukotrienes, prostaglandin D2, and platelet-activating factor are also released in response to mast cell activation [14].

Symptoms generally occur within seconds to minutes of starting the transfusion. On rare occasions, symptoms may take several hours to develop. It is important to distinguish symptoms associated with a transfusion-associated allergic reaction from a vasovagal response that can manifest with hypotension diaphoresis, nausea, vomiting, weakness, bradycardia, and occasionally loss of consciousness. In addition, patients who are taking angiotensin-converting enzyme (ACE) inhibitors may develop an isolated hypotension. This is thought to occur due to the dual actions on bradykinin caused both by the inhibition of catabolism by the ACE inhibitor and the activation of prekallikrein activity in the plasma protein fraction.

Premedication with antihistamines, approximately 30 min before transfusion, may help to prevent allergic reactions. If antihistamines are not sufficient, premedicating with prednisone or parenteral steroids may be useful. If premedication does not work, washing red cells or platelets prior to transfusion may be of some benefit. In patients who develop urticaria, the transfusion should be paused in order to administer diphenhydramine. A mild allergic reaction is the only transfusion reaction scenario in which administration of the remainder of the blood component may be resumed after treatment, and no laboratory investigation is required. Severe urticarial reactions may require treatment with methylprednisolone. If, however, symptoms do not subside or are accompanied by more severe symptoms such as hypotension or dyspnea, the transfusion must then be stopped. The patient's hypotension can be treated by placing them in the Trendelenburg position and infusing them with crystalloids. In cases of suspected anaphylaxis, prompt efforts should be made to maintain the airway and provide oxygenation. Epinephrine may be used in this case, with doses being repeated every 5–15 min up to three times unless palpitations, anxiousness, or tremors develop. If bronchospasm does not respond to epinephrine, the addition of a beta II agonist or aminophylline may be required. Patients who are unresponsive due to an ACE inhibitor or beta-adrenergic blocker may respond to intravenous glucagon [4]. In addition, patients with anaphylaxis should be tested for antibodies against immunoglobulin A (anti-IgA), and quantitative IgA levels should be assessed. In patients who are found to have an IgA deficiency, they should subsequently be transfused with components from IgA-deficient donors or after cellular components have been washed.

Hypothermia

Neonates are particularly susceptible to the life-threatening side effects of hypothermia, due to their decreased body fat, an immature epidermal barrier, and higher surface area to weight ratio [26, 38]. Complications of hypothermia can include alterations in pulmonary vasomotor tone, acid–base imbalances, an increased metabolic rate, hypoglycemia, and apnea leading to cardiac arrest. This is especially true during massive transfusions such as ECMO, exchange transfusions, cardiac surgery, and trauma. Even blood products at room temperature have been shown to decrease an infant's core body temperature by 0.7–2.5 C. Therefore, in-line blood warmers are required for all neonatal RBC exchange transfusions. It is important to remember, however, that heating blood products to elevated temperatures can cause red cell damage with associated increases in lactate dehydrogenase, extracellular potassium, and plasma hemoglobin due to hemolysis. Because of this, only FDA-approved devices that can accurately measure and maintain the temperate of the blood product should be used.

Transfusion-Related Acute Lung Injury

Transfusion-related acute lung injury (TRALI) is estimated to occur in 1 of every 1300–5000 transfusions and is the leading cause of transfusion-related mortality. All plasma-containing blood components, including whole blood, red blood cells, platelets, cryoprecipitate, and fresh frozen plasma, have been implicated in TRALI reactions with as little as 15 mL transfusion volumes. The symptoms of TRALI typically include fever, chills, dyspnea, cyanosis, hypotension, and the new onset of bilateral pulmonary edema [54]. Symptoms generally occur within hours of transfusion and can be fatal. The lung injury that occurs with TRALI is defined as hypoxemia with a PaO2/FiO2 ratio of 300 mmHg, radiographic evidence of bilateral pulmonary edema, no preexisting acute lung injury present before the transfusion occurred, onset of symptoms within 6 h of transfusion, and no temporal relationship to alternative risk factors for acute lung injury. TRALI can often be confused with acute respiratory distress syndrome (ARDS). However, where ARDS is often irreversible, TRALI is often transient. The majority of patients will show improvement after 48–96 h despite the need for mechanical ventilation and oxygen supplementation. Most commonly, TRALI is confused with transfusion-associated circulatory overload (TACO), where pulmonary edema is seen but is a result of cardiogenic factors. Unfortunately, up to 20 % of patients with TRALI will experience either a prolonged clinical course or even death.

While the exact mechanism is unknown, TRALI has been associated with antibodies to leukocyte antigens and the transfusion of biologic response modifiers (BRMs) [55, 64] that initiate a sequence of events resulting in cellular activation, basement membrane damage, and leakage of protein-rich fluid into alveolar spaces leading to pulmonary edema. A two-event model has been proposed as the mechanism of TRALI [65]. The first event occurs when biologically active compounds activate pulmonary vascular endothelial cells and prime neutrophils resulting in the sequestration of neutrophils within the pulmonary vasculature. In addition to transfusion, this first event can occur in sepsis and after surgery, therefore predisposing the patient to developing TRALI. The second event occurs when BRMs or antibodies are transfused into the recipient's circulation and activate the primed neutrophils within the pulmonary microvasculature. This results in pulmonary endothelial damage, capillary leakage, and pulmonary edema. In the majority of cases, the source of the antibodies is the donor rather than the recipient. Specifically, antibodies to HLA class I antigens, HLA class II antigens, and human neutrophil antigens (HNAs) have been implicated in TRALI which can form after exposure to foreign antigens during pregnancy, prior transfusions, or transplantation.

In patients with TRALI, treatment consists of respiratory and circulatory support including oxygen supplementation, possible mechanical ventilation, and pressors to support blood pressure. Unlike TACO, diuretics are unnecessary in TRALI because the associated pulmonary edema is not a result of circulatory overload. In addition, corticosteroids have been shown to improve clinical outcomes [68].

Methods to help prevent TRALI reactions include the use of male-donor or nulliparous female-donor plasma exclusively for transfusions while diverting multiparous female-donor plasma for fractionation as the prevalence of HLA antibodies increases with each subsequent pregnancy and testing female-plasma donors for the presence of HLA antibodies. These measures do not address this issue of antibodies to HNAs, however. Directed donations from blood relatives, particularly the mother, should also be discouraged as TRALI has been reported in this donor population [5, 7, 18, 75]. In cases of suspected TRALI, a sample of the donor's serum should be tested for the presence of HLA and HNA antibodies. Also, HLA typing the patient will help confirm TRALI cases, if in fact the donor has the corresponding HLA antibody to the patient's HLA antigens.

Transfusion-Associated Circulatory Overload

Transfusion-associated circulatory overload (TACO) has been estimated to occur in approximately 1 in 700 red blood cell recipients, with up to 20% of these patients having received only a single unit. TACO also accounts for 8% of transfusion-associated fatalities. TACO generally occurs within 1–2 h of transfusion and is associated with jugular venous distension, gallop, elevated central venous pressure, dyspnea, orthopnea, new ST segment or T wave changes on electrocardiogram, elevated serum troponins, and increased blood pressure with a widening of the pulse pressure. Imaging often shows a widened cardiothoracic ratio. While large transfusion volumes and high flow rates are frequently implicated in TACO, volume overload has been seen even with modest transfusion volumes.

TACO is often confused for TRALI due to the fact that they both present with pulmonary edema. It is, of course, possible for a patient to develop both TACO and TRALI after a transfusion. However, TACO can be differentiated based on the presence of hypertension and rapid improvement with either diuretics or inotropic agents. In addition, laboratory studies showing a pre-transfusion to post-transfusion brain natriuretic peptide ratio of 1.5 with a posttransfusion level of greater than 100 pg/mL have an 80% sensitivity and specificity level for TACO.

As soon as TACO is suspected, the transfusion should be stopped, and the patient should be placed in the seated position. Supplemental oxygen should be administered as needed, and the patient should be placed on diuretics in order to reduce the intravascular volume. If symptoms persist in confirmed TACO, additional diuretics of therapeutic phlebotomy may be utilized. While the majority of neonates do not benefit from volume reduction due to platelet loss during centrifugation, concentrating or volume-reducing platelets helps to minimize the risk of volume overload. Patients at risk for volume overload include infants with cardiac diseases and oliguric renal failure. However, concentration performed using an open system procedure limits the shelf life to 4 h. Also, concentration can activate platelets during centrifugation, and the pH of concentrated platelets stored in a syringe rapidly declines and should therefore be transfused as soon as possible.

Transfusion-Associated Necrotizing Enterocolitis

Necrotizing enterocolitis (NEC) is a common yet devastating condition in neonates which carries significant morbidity and mortality and very few treatment options. NEC is estimated to effect between 6 and 10% of very-low-birth-weight (<1500 g) infants and leads to an increased length of hospital stay [45]. The etiology of NEC is multifactorial with risk factors including prematurity, small for gestational age, hypoxic-ischemic events, early and rapid advancements of enteral feeds, formula feeds, bacterial overgrowth, and even exposure to platelet-activating factor acetylhydrolase present in platelet suspensions [20]. The prevalence of NEC is estimated to be 5%.

While some studies did not find recent red blood cell transfusion to be a risk factor for developing NEC [32, 62], others have suggested the potential role of red blood cell transfusions in causing what is known as transfusion-associated NEC (TANEC) [21]. Although the exact mechanism is unclear, some have proposed theories include an underlying medical condition; extreme anemia with impaired blood flow to the gastrointestinal system; altered blood flow during feeding; exposure to biologically active mediators such as free hemoglobin, increased cytokines, and broken red cell fragments within the transfused blood which triggers an immunologic response within the intestinal mucosa; altered angiogenesis within the intestine; and reperfusion associated with transfusion [2, 52]. Studies have shown that infants who develop TANEC tend to be younger, lower birth weight, have higher illness severity scores, have a patent ductus arteriosus with intestinal "steal" [22], be receiving ventilator support [42], and have exposure to transfusion within 48 h when compared to infants with NEC not associated with transfusion [70]. While the risk factors may differ, some studies have shown that there are little differences in morbidity or mortality between infants with TANEC and those with NEC not associated with transfusion [70]. In contrast, other studies suggest that TANEC is associated with an increased need for surgical intervention [52], prolonged hospitalization [30], and increased mortality [6, 41] than those with NEC not associated with transfusion. It is important to note that the factors that place neonates at increased risk for TANEC (i.e., prematurity, low birth weight, etc.) are all independently associated with adverse outcomes and may be confounding.

Some proposed suggestions in reducing the occurrence of TANEC include withholding feeds during the transfusion in order to counteract postprandial alterations in blood flow. In addition, bacteria from the gastrointestinal tract release sialidases which are enzymes that cleave sialic acid residues creating neonatigens. Naturally occurring complement-dependent antibodies can cause lysis of the neoantigen-labeled red blood cells. T activation in infants is common (approximately 13 % of infants in NICU), while hemolysis is less common. Therefore, it is controversial as to whether it is necessary to provide washed red cells to all neonates with necrotizing enterocolitis or only those with evidence of hemolysis.

T Activation and Positive Lectins

Several case reports have identified hemolysis after the transfusion of blood products in infants, generally occurring in association with NEC. It has been suggested that this hemolysis occurs as a result of T activation, which refers to alterations in RBC membrane glycoprotein structure generally by microbial enzymatic action. The T antigen, an exposed RBC cryptantigen, binds to the IgM anti-T [56] which leads to the removal of N-acetylneuraminic acid (also known as sialic acid) from the RBC by neuraminidase [27]. Anti-T is present in the plasma of most adults but is generally absent in early infancy [43]. It is believed that many bacteria and viruses contain a substance that is identical to the T antigen [67]. Because of this, antibodies are formed as a result of antigenic stimulation by intestinal flora in a manner similar to the development of ABO antibodies. Neuraminidase is produced by many microbiologic agents including bacteria, viruses, and protozoa. In addition, neuraminidase-producing organisms are known to produce hemolytic toxins as well [43]. T antigen activation has also been reported in association with anaerobic, especially clostridial, sepsis, and other severe infections. Animal studies have suggested that hemolysis of T-activated RBCs is due to the enhanced clearance of RBCs containing decreased N-acetylneuraminic acid rather than immunologic-mediated mechanisms [15, 19].

Variants of T activation, including Th and Tx activation, occur less commonly and are thought to be incomplete forms of T activation [27, 56]. Tk and Tn activation, however, are different and distinct from T activation. Tk activation occurs due to exposure to N-acetylglucosamine by the bacterial enzyme β-galactosidase which cleaves the terminal galactose residue from the RBC. In contrast, Tn is not induced by microbial action but rather results from a clonal RBC mutation that is persistent rather than transient [3]. In order to distinguish between the various types of polyagglutinable RBCs, testing can be performed with a panel of lectins. Table 6.1 identifies the major lectins and their reactions with different erythrocyte cryptoantigens involved in polyagglutination.

Because of the severe hemolysis that can occur following the transfusion of blood products in infants with T-activated RBCs, many clinicians avoid or delay the transfusion of plasma-containing blood components to neonates who are at high risk of T activations, particularly those with NEC [33, 47]. Therefore, the routine screening of infant RBCs for T activation, ensuring the availability of low-titer anti-T blood com-

Table 6.1 Major lectins and reactivity with erythrocyte crypoantigens

Lectins	Erythrocyte cryptoantigens				
	T	Tk	Tn	Cad	Tx
Arachis hypogaea	+	+	−	−	+
Dolichos biflorus	−	−	+	+	−
Glycine soja	+	−	+	+	−
Salvia sclarea	−	−	+	−	−
Salvia horminum	−	−	+w	+	−
Bandeiraea simplicifolia	−	+	−	−	−
Salvia farinacea	−	−	+w	+	−
Leonurus cardiaca	−	−	−	+	−
Vicia cretica	+	−	−	−	−
Medicago disciformis	+	−	−	−	−

ponents, and washing plasma-containing blood components in lectin-positive patients has been considered. However, one study found that although infants with T and T variant-activated RBCs had a higher rate of hemolysis and mortality, the use of low-titer anti-T blood products did not reduce the rate of mortality [49]. In addition, the washing of blood products could lead to a delay in appropriate treatment, thereby putting the patient at risk. Currently, there is no expert consensus, and additional studies are warranted to implement changes in clinical practice.

Transfusion-Associated Graft-Versus-Host Disease

Transfusion-associated graft-versus-host disease (TA-GVHD) is a rare complication of blood transfusion. TA-GVHD occurs when donor lymphocytes from transfused blood mount an immune response against the recipient. A key mechanism in TA-GVHD is the inability of the host's immune system to recognize or fight off the donor cells transferred via transfusion. TA-GVHD most frequently occurs in immunocompromised patients. Given their immature immune system, neonatal patients are at particular risk for developing TA-GVHD. However, TA-GVHD can also occur in immunocompetent patients with no underlying diagnosis known to cause immune compromise. This may occur with shared HLA antigens when the donor lymphocytes are able to evade the host immune response. Rarely, TA-GVHD has been associated with extreme prematurity, neonatal alloimmune thrombocytopenia, and extracorporeal membrane oxygenation (ECMO).

One study found that the majority of cases of TA-GVHD occurred after transfusion of cellular components less than 10 days old that were not leukoreduced and not irradiated [36]. The number of lymphocytes present within a donor sample may also play a role in TA-GVHD, with a significant reduction in the risk of developing TA-GVHD occurring after leukoreduction. Neonatal patients with TA-GVHD typically present with fever, rash, gastrointestinal symptoms, liver injury, and hypoproliferative pancytopenia. The diagnosis of TA-GVHD can be made based on a combination of characteristic clinical findings, tissue biopsy, and leukocyte chimerism (the presence of donor lymphocytes in recipient tissue) occurring between 2 days to 6 weeks after receiving a transfusion. It is recommended that any patient exhibiting signs and symptoms of TA-GVHD receives a thorough evaluation and workup including investigation of HLA antigens.

Unfortunately, TA-GVHD is associated with >90% mortality and has limited treatment options. However, TA-GVHD can be prevented with pre-transfusion irradiation of blood products. As previously mentioned, new photochemical pathogen inactivation treatments have been shown to be effective at inactivating bacteria, viruses, protozoa, and donor leukocyte contaminants within plasma and platelet units while preserving to therapeutic effectiveness of the blood component and may also help to prevent TA-GVHD.

References

1. Andreu G, Morel P, Forestier F, et al. Hemovigilance network in France: organization and analysis of immediate transfusion incidence reports from 1994 to 1998. Transfusion. 2002;42:1356–64.
2. Blau J, Calo JM, Dozor D, et al. Transfusion-related acute gut injury: necrotizing enterocolitis in very low birth weight neonates after packed red blood cell transfusion. J Pediatr. 2011;158(3):403–9.
3. Boralessa H, Modi N, Cockburn H, et al. RBC T activation and hemolysis in a neonatal intensive care population: implications for transfusion practice. Transfusion. 2002;42:1428–34.
4. Brown SGA, Mullins RJ, Gold MS. Anaphylaxis: diagnosis and management. Med J Aust. 2006;185:283–9.
5. Campbell Jr DA, Swartz RD, Waskerwitz JA, et al. Leukoagglutiniation with interstitial pulmonary edema. A complication of donor-specific transfusion. Transplantation. 1982;34:300–1.
6. Christensen RD, Lambert DK, Henry E, et al. Is "transfusion-associated necrotizing enterocolitis" an authentic pathogenic entity? Transfusion. 2010;31(3):183–7.
7. Church GD, Price C, Sanchez R, et al. Transfusion-related acute lung injury in the paediatric patient: two case reports and a review of the literature. Transfus Med. 2006;16:343–8.
8. Ciaravino V, Hanover J, Lin L, Sullivan T, Corash L. Assessment of safety in neonates for transfusion of platelets and plasma prepared with amotosalen photochemical pathogen inactivation treatment by a 1-month intravenous toxicity study in neonatal rats. Transfusion. 2009;49:985–94.
9. Ciaravino V, McCullough T, Cimino G, Sullivan T, et al. Preclinical safety profile of plasma prepared using the INTERCEPT blood system. Vox Sang. 2003;85:171–82.
10. Ciaravino V, McCullough T, Cimino G. The role of toxicology assessment in transfusion medicine. Transfusion. 2003;43:1481–92.
11. Collard KJ. Is there a causal relationship between the receipt of blood transfusions and and the development of chronic lung disease of prematurity? Med Hypotheses. 2006;66:355–64.
12. Cooke RWI, Clark D, Hickey-Dwyer M, et al. The apparent role of blood transfusions in the development of retinopathy of prematurity. Eur J Pediatr. 1993;152:833–6.
13. Cooke RW, Drury JA, Yoxall CW, et al. Blood transfusion and chronic lung disease in preterm infants. Eur J Pediatr. 1997;156:47–50.
14. Cotran RS, editor. Robbins pathologic basis of disease. 9th ed. Philipdelphia: WB Saunders; 2014. p. 178.
15. Crookston KP, Reiner AP, Cooper LJN, et al. RBC T-activation and hemolysis: implications for pediatric transfusion management. Transfusion. 2000;40:801–12.
16. Davenport RD. Hemolytic transfusion reactions. In: Popovsky MA, editor. Transfusion reactions. 3rd ed. Bethesda: AABB Press; 2007. p. 1–55.
17. Domen RE, Hoeltge GA. Allergic transfusion reactions: an evaluation of 273 consecutive reactions. Arch Pathol Lab Med. 2003;127:316–20.
18. Dunbar N, Cooke M, Diab M, Toy P. Transfusion-related acute lung injury after transfusion of maternal blood: a case–control study. Spine. 2010;35(23):1322–7.
19. Durocher JR, Payne RC, Conrad ME. Role of sialic acid in erythrocyte survival. Blood. 1975;45:11–20.
20. Furukawa M, Lee EL, Johnston JM. Platelet-activating factor-induced ischemic bowel necrosis: the effect of platelet-activating factor acetylhydrolase. Pediatr Res. 1993;34:237–41.
21. Garg PM, Ravisankar S, Bian H, Macgilvray S, Shekhawat P. Relationship between packed red blood cell transfusion and severe form of necrotizing enterocolitis: a case control study. Indian Pediatr. 2015;52:1041–5.
22. Gupta S, Wylie J, and Plews D. Hemodynamic effects of packed red blood cell transfusion volume in premature infants: results of a randomized controlled trial. E-PAS. 2007;5899.6

23. Hall TL, Barnes A, Miller JR, et al. Neonatal mortality following transfusion of red cells with high plasma potassium levels. Transfusion. 1993;33:606–9.
24. Hebert PC, Wells G, Tweeddale M, et al. Does transfusion practice affect mortality in critically ill patients? Transfusion requirements in critical care (TRICC) investigators and the Canadian critical care trials group. Am J Respir Crit Care Med. 1997;155:1618–23.
25. Hennino A, Berard F, Guillot I, et al. Pathophysiology of urticaria. Clin Rev Allergy Immunol. 2006;30:3–11.
26. Horan M, Edwards AD, Firmin RK, et al. The effect of temperature on the QTc interval in the newborn infant receiving extracorporeal membrane oxygenation (ECMO). Early Hum Dev. 2007;83:217–23.
27. Horn KD. The classification, recognition and significance of polyagglutination in transfusion medicine. Blood Rev. 1999;13:36–44.
28. Josephson CD, Mullis NC, Van Demark C, et al. Significant numbers of apheresis-derived group O platelet units have "high-titer" anti-A/A, B: implications for transfusion policy. Transfusion. 2004;44:805–8.
29. Josephson CD, Su LL, et al. Platelet transfusion practice among neonatologists in the United States and Canada: results of a survey. Pediatrics. 2009;123:278–85.
30. Josephson CD, Wesolowski A, Bao G, et al. Do red cell transfusions increase the risk of necrotizing enterocolitis in premature infants? J Pediatr. 2010;157(6):972–8, e1–e3.
31. Kahn DJ, Richardson DK, Billett HH. Associated of thrombocytopenia and delivery method with intraventricular hemorrhage among very-low-birth-weight infants. Am K Obstet Gynecol. 2002;186(1):109–16.
32. Kirpalani H, Zupancic JA. Do transfusions cause necrotizing enterocolitis? The complementary role of randomized trials and observational studies. Semin Perinatol. 2012;36:269–76.
33. Klein RL, Novak RW, Novak PE. T-cryptantigen exposure in neonatal necrotizing enterocolitis. J Pediatr Surg. 1986;21:1155–8.
34. Knutson F, Osselaer J, Pierelli L, et al. A prospective, active haemovigilance study with combined cohort analysis of 19,175 transfusions of platelet components prepared with amotosalen-UVA photochemical treatment. Vox Sang. 2015;12287:1–10.
35. Kohn DJ, Richardson DK, Billett HH. Inter-NICU variation in rates and management of thrombocytopenia among very low birth-weight infants. J Perinatol. 2003;23(4):312–6.
36. Kopolovic I, Ostro J, Tsubota H, et al. A systematic review of transfusion-associated graft-versus-host disease. Blood. 2015;126:406–14.
37. Lambin P, Pennec L, Hauptmann G, et al. Adverse transfusion reactions associated with a precipitating anti-C4 antibody of anti-Rogers specificity. Vox Sang. 1984;47:242–9.
38. Laptook AR, Salhab W, Bhaskar B. Admission temperature of low birth weight infants: predictors and associated morbidities. Pediatrics. 2007;119:e643–9.
39. Levy G, Strauss R, Hume H, et al. National survey of neonatal transfusion practices: I. Red blood cell therapy. Pediatrics. 1993;91:523–9.
40. Luban N. Neonatal red blood cell transfusions. Cur Opin Hematol. 2002;9:533–6.
41. Mally P, Golombek SG, Mishra R, et al. Association of necrotizing enterocolitis with elective packed red blood cell transfusions in stable, growing, premature neonates. Am J Perinatol. 2006;23(8):451–8.
42. Mohamed A, Shah PS. Transfusion associated necrotizing enterocolitis: a meta-analysis of observational data. Pediatrics. 2012;129:529–40.
43. Mollison PL, Engelfriet CP, Contreras M, editors. Blood transfusion in clinical medicine. 10th ed. Oxford: Blackwell Scientific; 1997. p. 233–6.
44. Neonatal Transfusion Guidance. American Association of Blood Bankers. Revised 2012.
45. Neu J, Walker WA. Necrotizing enterocolitis. N Engl J Med. 2011;364:255–64.
46. New HV. Pediatric transfusion. Vox Sang. 2006;90:1–9.
47. Novak RW, Abbott AE, Klein RL. T-cryptantigen determination affects mortality in necrotizing enterocolitis. Surg Gynecol Obstet. 1993;176:368–70.
48. Ohls RK, Kamath-Rayne BD, et al. Cognitive outcomes of preterm infants randomized to darbepoetin, erythropoietin, or placebo. Pediatrics. 2014;133:1023–30.

49. Osborn DA, Lui K, Pussell P, et al. T and Tk antigen activation in necrotizing enterocolitis: manifestations, severity of illness, and effectiveness of testing. Arch Dis Child Fetal Neonatal Ed. 1999;80:F192–7.

50. Osselaer JC, Cazenave JP, Lambermont M, et al. An active hemovigilance program characterizing the safety profile of 7437 platelet transfusions prepared with amotosalen photochemical treatment. Vox Sang. 2008;94(4):315–23.

51. Osselaer JC, Messe N, Hervig T, et al. A prospective observational cohort safety study of 5106 platelet transfusions with components prepared with photochemical pathogen inactivation treatment. Transfusion. 2008;48(6):1061–71.

52. Paul DA, Mackley A, Novitsky A, et al. Increased odds of necrotizing enterocolitis after transfusions or red blood cells in premature infants. Pediatrics. 2011;127(4):635–41.

53. Pineda AA, Zylstra VW, Clare DE, et al. Viability and functional integrity of washed platelets. Transfusion. 1989;29:524–7.

54. Popovsky MA, Haley NR. Further characterization of transfusion-related acute lung injury: demographics, clinical and laboratory features and morbidity. Immunohematology. 2000;16:157–9.

55. Popovsky MA, Moore SB. Diagnostic and pathogenic considerations in transfusion-related acute lung injury. Transfusion. 1985;25:573–7.

56. Ramasethu J, Luban N. T-activation. Br J Haematol. 2001;112:259–63.

57. Roback JD, Grossman BJ, Harris T, Hillyer CD, editors. AABB Technical manual. 17th ed. Bethesda: AABB; 2011.

58. Sacks LM, Schaffer D, Anday EK, et al. Retrolental fibroplasia and blood transfusion in very low-birthweight infants. Pediatrics. 1981;68:770–4.

59. Sandler SG, Mallory D, Malamut D, et al. IgA anaphylactic transfusion reactions. Transfus Med Rev. 1995;9:1–8.

60. Sapatnekar S, Sharma G, Downes KA, et al. AHTR in a pediatric patient following transfusion of apheresis platelets. J Clin Apher. 2005;20:225–9.

61. Schoenfeld H, Muhm M, Doepfmer U, et al. Platelet activity in washed platelet concentrations. Anesth Analg. 2004;99:17–20.

62. Sharma R, Kraemer DF, Torrazza RM, Mai V, et al. Packed red blood cell transfusion is not associated with increased risk of necrotizing enterocolitis in premature infants. J Perinatol. 2014;34:858–62.

63. Shimada E, Odagiri M, Chaiwong K, et al. Detection of Hp(del) among Thais, a deleted allele of the haptoglobin gene that causes congenital haptoglobin deficiency. Transfusion. 2007;47:2315–21.

64. Silliman CC, Ambruso DR, Boshkov LK. Transfusion-related acute lung injury. Blood. 2005;105:2266–73.

65. Silliman CC, Boshkov LK, Mehdizadehkashi Z, et al. Transfusion-related acute lung injury: epidemiology and a prospective analysis of etiologic factors. Blood. 2003;101:452–62.

66. Slonim AD, Joseph JG, Turenne WM, et al. Blood transfusions in children: a multi-institutional analysis of practices and complications. Transfusion. 2008;48:73–80.

67. Springer GF, Tegtmeyer H. Origin of anti-Thomsen-Friedenreich (T) and Tn agglutinins in man and in White Leghorn chicks. Br J Haematol. 1981;47:453–60.

68. Steinberg KP, Hudson LD, Goodman RB, et al. Efficacy and safety of corticosteroids for persistent acute respiratory distress syndrome. N Engl J Med. 2006;354:1671–84.

69. Strauss RG. Transfusion therapy in neonates. Am J Dis Child. 1991;145:904–11.

70. Stritzke AI, Smyth J, Synnes A, et al. Transfusion-associated necrotizing enterocolitis in neonates. Arch Dis Child Fetal Neonatal Ed. 2012. doi:10.1136/fetalneonatal-2011-301282.

71. Sullivan MT, McCullough J, Schreiber GB, et al. Blood collection and transfusion in the United States in 1997. Transfusion. 2002;42:1253–60.

72. Vamvakas EC. Allergic and anaphylactic reactions. In: Popovsky MA, editor. Transfusion reactions. 3rd ed. Bethesda: AABB Press; 2007. p. 105–56.

73. Vamvakas EC, Blajchman MA. Transfusion-related mortality: the ongoing risks of allogeneic blood transfusion and the available strategies for their prevention. Blood. 2009;113:3406–17.

74. Wollowitz S. Fundamentals of the psoralen-based Helinx technology for inactivation of infectious pathogens and leukocytes in platelets and plasma. Semin Hematol. 2001;38 Suppl 11:4–11.
75. Yang X, Ahmed S, Chandrasekaran V. Transfusion-related acute lung injury resulting from designated blood transfusion between mother and child: a report of two cases. Am J Clin Pathol. 2004;121:590–2.

Chapter 7
Transfusion Considerations for Neonatal Extracorporeal Membrane Oxygenation (ECMO)

Ursula Nawab and Susan B. Williams

ECMO

In 1976, Baby Esperanza (Spanish for "hope"), the first successful neonatal case of ECMO, brought babies a new "hope" for survival and a future that was not possible a decade earlier. Dr. Bartlett took cardiopulmonary bypass to the bedside ushering in a new therapy for the most critical neonates. Physiologically reversible diseases requiring time for neonates to transition but with no means of supporting their cardio/respiratory failure experienced now had a therapeutic option. Instead of almost certain mortality, Bartlett et al. described >50 % survival. A new treatment was born, essentially creating a supportive intensive care therapy for acute, reversible cardio/respiratory failure. ECMO (extracorporeal membrane oxygenation) is a complex, expensive, invasive procedure requiring the expertise of many to save one. Because ECMO requires a multidisciplinary

U. Nawab (✉)
Department of Pediatrics, Division of Neonatology,
The Children's Hospital of Philadelphia, Perelman School of
Medicine University of Pennsylvania, Philadelphia, PA, USA
e-mail: NAWABU@email.chop.edu

S.B. Williams, RN, BSW, RNC-NIC
ECMO Center, The Children's Hospital of Philadelphia,
34th Street and Civic Center Blvd., 2NW66 Main Hospital,
Philadelphia, PA, USA
e-mail: williamssu@email.chop.edu

© Springer International Publishing Switzerland 2017
D.A. Sesok-Pizzini (ed.), *Neonatal Transfusion Practices*,
DOI 10.1007/978-3-319-42764-5_7

103

team and a range of consultative services (including neonatology, pediatric surgery, neurology, cardiology, critical care nurses, respiratory therapists, ECMO specialists, perfusionists, and transfusion services), critically ill neonates require transfer to tertiary care hospitals for this care. Babies are placed on partial cardiopulmonary bypass to support respiratory and cardiac function. With the focus on maintaining adequate oxygenation while allowing time for the intrinsic recovery of the heart and lungs, ECMO can be used to support patients for days to weeks. It provides long-term cardiorespiratory support in neonates with a high likelihood of dying when standard medical therapy has failed [4].

Since Bartlett's first reports of survival in the early 1980s, neonates have seen significant improvement in survival outcomes [27]. In 2013, 68 % of all infants receiving ECMO survive [46]. Evaluating respiratory morbidities alone, survival is 75 %, while complex cardiac diseases and ECPR demonstrate a 40 % survival. Despite advances in medical therapy, ECMO remains an effective treatment for neonatal respiratory failure [36] yielding good cognitive and functional outcomes as well as improved long-term morbidities [10]. Over the past decade, it has been used on increasing complex and acutely ill babies for days to weeks to months.

Description (VA Versus VV)

ECMO is a modified cardiopulmonary bypass where venous blood is directed to a circuit (pump and oxygenator), oxygenated, and then returned to the body via a major blood vessel (artery or vein). ECMO is achieved via extrathoracic cannulation of cervical vessels with two modes of support: venoarterial (VA) providing cardiac and respiratory support and venovenous (VV) supplying respiratory support alone.

VA ECMO, the primary ECMO procedure performed through the years, is most commonly used to date. During VA ECMO, cannulae are placed in the right common carotid artery and internal jugular vein. The tip of the venous catheter is advanced into the right atrium, while the arterial catheter is positioned at the junction of the right common carotid artery into the aortic arch, requiring ligation of the distal right carotid artery [31]. Once on bypass, venous blood is actively pumped through the oxygenator where gas exchange occurs. The blood is then warmed to body temperature by the heat exchanger and then returned to the body via the right carotid artery. Because there is complete bypass of the heart, VA ECMO provides both cardiac and pulmonary support and is the method of choice for patients with severe blood pressure instability or primary cardiac dysfunction. Although providing direct circulatory support, VA ECMO causes an increase in left ventricular afterload which coupled with hypoxic coronary perfusion from desaturated blood in the left ventricle may result in cardiac stun. "Stun" is a state of exaggerated decrease or absence of ventricular/myocardial performance. VA ECMO is associated with an increase in long-term neurological complications [2].

VV ECMO, the preferred mode of ECMO for appropriate candidates with adequate cardiac function, has increased over the past decade [4]. A double-lumen catheter is placed through the right internal jugular vein into the right atrium. Desaturated blood is drained from the right atrium via the outer fenestrated port and returned by the inner second port angled to direct blood flow across the tricuspid valve. Single-site VV only requires cannulation of the right internal jugular vein and does not involve manipulation or ligation of an arterial structure. VV ECMO is greatly dependent on the degree of venous return to the circuit. The use of a cephalad catheter, a single-lumen cannula placed in the cephalad part of the right internal jugular vein, can help augment venous return, allowing for cerebral venous decompression and reducing recirculation [45]. As blood flow is returned to the right side of the heart, VV ECMO does not provide direct circulatory support and requires innate myocardial performance. As a result of recirculation, it may not achieve the same degree of systemic oxygenation as VA ECMO. However, despite the lack of circulatory support, myocardial performance may indirectly be improved by pulmonary vasodilation from the mixed venous saturations coupled with decreased left ventricular afterload leading to improve coronary perfusion. VV ECMO has been associated with increased survival and a shorter duration of ECMO [2].

ECMO Circuit

The ECMO circuit is designed to mechanically support a baby for a prolonged duration of time from days to weeks. It principally provides mechanical organs which function as circulatory and respiratory systems, pumping blood through an artificial lung which removes carbon dioxide and adds oxygen and returning warmed blood to the patient. The basics of the ECMO circuit consist of a blood pump, a gas exchange device/oxygenator, and a heat exchanger connected with conduit tubing [33]. In the modern circuits, there are built-in sensors for safety and monitoring. These additional features include a pressure monitor to assess for thrombosis or occlusion of the tubing, venous oxygen saturation monitor to assess global perfusion, and a temperature monitor for the heat exchanger to maintain adequate patient temperatures.

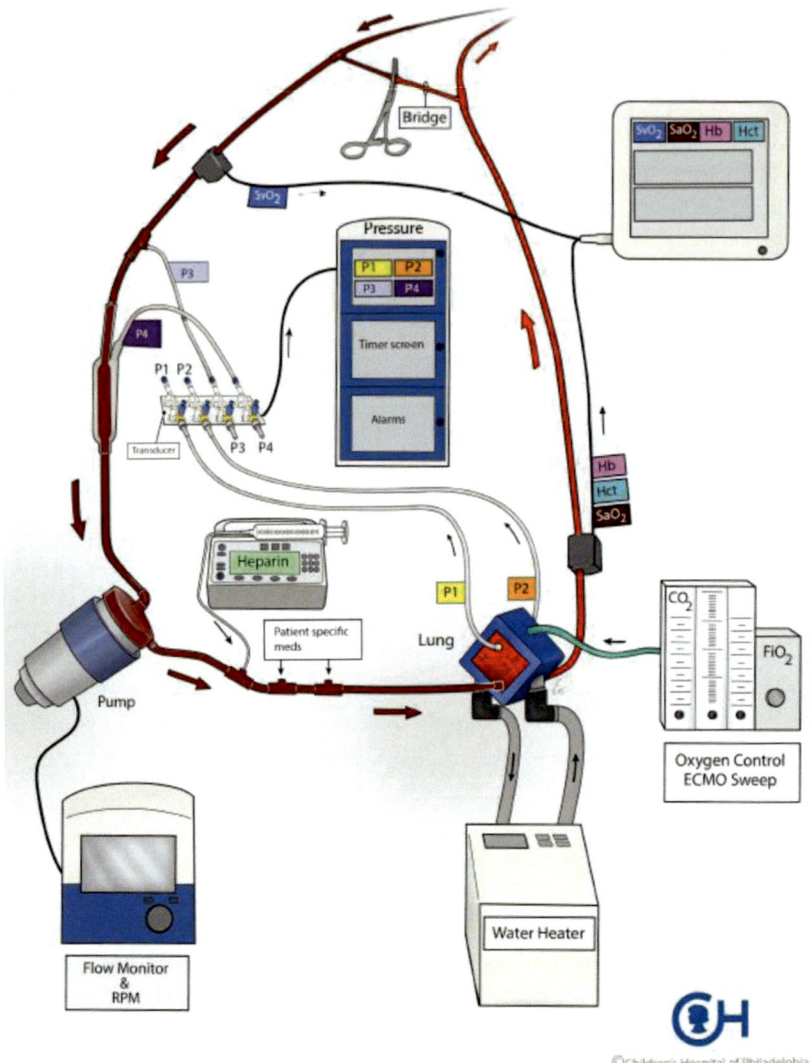

Bladder/Reservoir

Blood flows from the cannula via gravity into this chamber which serves to regulate flow through the pump and oxygenator. It acts as the gauge pump flow through a servoregulation mechanism controlling the pump. If venous return is adequate, the bladder is distended and maintains pump flow rate. If negative pressures are generated secondary to decreased venous return, the bladder collapses and interrupts the pump flow minimizing the risk of cavitation (air being pulled into the circuit). In cases of low flow through the pump, there are risks of clot formation in apex and base of the bladder.

Pump

The pump is the "heart" of the circuit. Over the past decades, the standard for neonatal ECMO has been the semiocclusive roller pump which produces flow by displacing fluid with a direct and repeated pressure against a compressible tube. Due to active compression by an occlusive rotor, it is resistance independent and produces constant flow. Roller pumps function exceptionally well at the low flows typically used in neonates.

Recently, there has been an emergence of the centrifugal pump which is currently used in pediatrics and adult ECMO in many centers. A centrifugal pump converts rotational energy into kinetic energy dispersing fluid radially with a centrifugal force. It is a nonocclusive mechanism that is resistance dependent; therefore it is extremely sensitive to patient volume status (preload) and afterload. Modern centrifugal pumps are compact and require a small prime volume. At high flows, less mechanical energy is needed to move blood. However, high RPMs and excess heat generation can lead to shear stress on the red cells causing hemolysis, particularly in low-flow cases as seen in neonatal cases.

Due to these effects on the red blood cells at lower flow states, some have concerns with its use in neonatal ECMO. Masalunga et al. reported an increase in hemolysis in neonatal ECMO cases with the use of centrifugal vs. roller pumps [37] [6]. Additionally, Barrett et al. found increased risk of acute renal failure, hyperbilirubinemia, and need for inotropic support on ECMO [6, 49].

Oxygenator

The oxygenator acts as the "lung" of the circuit as it is the site of gas exchange. They can be made of a variety of materials from silicone to polymethylpentene to polypropylene. The classic lung was the silicone membrane lung which consisted of a flat sheet of silicone through which blood and gas flow in countercurrent directions. Currently, a polymethylpentene diffusion membrane (PMP) lung is being utilized across centers. The PMP consists of hollow fibers protected by a thin outer layer which acts as the site of gas transfer. In both the silicone lung and the PMP, gas exchange occurs through diffusion across these surfaces.

Heat Exchanger

With the large surface area of the circuit exposed to ambient temperature and a flow equivalent to the cardiac output of a neonate going through the circuit, the risk of hypothermia is significant. While a heat exchanger is not necessarily required for CPB time-limited cases in the OR, it is a vital component to the ECMO circuit in the neonate as it mitigates the ambient heat loss and maintains normothermia.

ECMO for Respiratory Failure

The initial cases of neonatal ECMO were in babies with respiratory failure who were not successfully transitioning from in utero circulation. Table 7.1 includes the most common diagnoses requiring ECMO.

There are no universally accepted criteria for initiation of ECMO. When the initial entry criteria were created, it was based on selecting infants with the highest projected mortality. While there is slight variation, most centers currently exclude cases secondary to prematurity, lethal or irreversible conditions, or limitations of equipment/technology (e.g., cannula size) (see Table 7.2).

Table 7.1 Indications

Respiratory	Cardiac
Meconium aspiration syndrome	Inadequate cardiac output and end-organ injury refractory to medical therapy
Congenital diaphragmatic hernia (CDH)	Preoperative stabilization
Sepsis	Failure to separate from cardiopulmonary bypass
Persistent pulmonary hypertension of the newborn	Postcardiotomy low cardiac output states
Respiratory distress syndrome	Bridge to transplantation
Congenital lung abnormalities	Single-ventricle heart disease
Hypoxic respiratory failure refractory to medical therapy	Cardiomyopathy
	Myocarditis
	Pulmonary hypertension
	Intractable dysrhythmia
	Cardiac arrest
	Low cardiac output states unrelated to structural heart disease

Table 7.2 Contraindications

Absolute	Relative
Grade III or greater ICH	Birth weight <1.6 kg
Severe irreversible brain damage	Gestational age <34 weeks
Lethal malformations or lethal congenital anomalies	Irreversible organ damage (unless considered for organ transplant)
	Disease states with a high probability of poor prognosis: Uncorrectable heart disease Preexisting coagulopathy or uncontrolled bleeding
	Ventilation with 100 % oxygen for ≥14 days

Annich et al. [4]

Over the years, the population meeting these criteria has demonstrated the most dramatic improvement in survival. It is now considered standard of care for neonates (term or late preterm) presenting with hypoxemic respiratory failure unresponsive to optimal medical management. The difficulty these days is in defining "failure to improve on other medical therapies" and deciding the most favorable timing of intervention [4]. Whereas in the past ECMO was considered a "last-ditch effort," currently the decision to cannulate is just as much about decreasing morbidity as it prevents mortality. Over the years, the ECMO population has shifted to more complex cases with higher acuity [46, 50].

Guidelines for Transfusion Support

Significant transfusion support is required for neonatal ECMO, and the presenting challenges are similar to that of trauma patients [62]. Urgency of the case determines what type of blood and how quick it should be prepared – immediate which is typically an unexpected case requiring rapid stabilization vs. standby cases which may occur in the near future. Communication with the primary team is paramount for safety and efficiency in preparing these cases – particularly in determining the preparation of products, location of procedure, and timing. Consent for blood products and specimen typing and screening must be considered prior to a procedure. The use of blood components and thus the role of the transfusion services are vital during ECMO as it is essentially a large-volume transfusion (transfusion of blood components equaling one or more blood volumes in a 24-h period) [15]. Blood product needs occur throughout the ECMO course, initially during priming and subsequently in ongoing support for routine circuit maintenance as well as emergent situations, such as acute hemorrhage or unanticipated disruptions of the circuit. The type of product, amount, and frequency of product use are dependent on a variety of clinical variables (i.e., diagnosis, duration of ECMO, and type of ECMO). Coordinated care between the primary service and transfusion service improves the care for these patients.

Priming

Whereas adult ECMO circuits are saline primed and ready for immediate use, the priming of the neonatal ECMO circuit requires some degree of preparation from transfusion services. Packed red cells are utilized in the priming secondary to the relatively large volumes required in a patient <10 k. Transient hypovolemia and hemodilution is not well tolerated in neonates and can lead to hemodynamic instability.

The neonatal circuit volume is 400–500 mL which is typically 1–2 times the blood volume of a neonate (80–90 ml/k) [58]. Care must be taken with priming considering the volume required as pH, hematocrit, calcium, coagulation, electrolytes, and temperature will be affected in the patient due to the blood prime. For this reason, the circuit is primed with the freshest blood for the theoretical benefits of lower potassium load, lower pH, and improved oxygen release from 2,3 DPG-enriched RBCs [43]. In the absence of fresh blood, saline-washed blood may be used though risk of hemolysis is slightly increased due to increased osmotic fragility of red cells [37].

Ideally, priming would consist of 1–2 units of ABO and Rh group-specific and crossmatch-compatible PRBCs with one unit of FFP. However, as ECMO occurs in critically ill neonates in situations where sufficient time for pre-transfusion testing may not occur, group O Rh (D)-negative red cell products and group AB plasma products can be used for ECMO circuit. To avoid hemodynamic instability and hemodilution caused by the standard saline circuit, the typical prime components include PRBCs, FFP, 25 % albumin, crystalloid, heparin, calcium gluconate, and NaHCO3. The hematocrit of the priming solution is 40–45 %.

Ongoing Transfusion Support

Transfusion support for this group is especially challenging. There must be a readily available supply of products throughout the ECMO course. Anemia secondary to hemolysis can develop. PRBCs are required for maintenance of the circuit. Complications related to bleeding may unexpectedly and acutely occur as well as the need for emergent circuit changes [62].

After initiation of ECMO, there is a 40–50 % drop in platelets and platelet inactivation coupled with activation and consumption of coagulation factors leading to variable degrees of coagulopathy [24]. Jackson et al. found over a 27-year period that the median blood product use was 36.2 mL/kg/day of PRBC and 8.1 mL/kg/day of platelets [26]. Transfusion requirements for an ECMO course are considerable regardless of the indication; however, surgical cases such as the cardiac and CDH populations tend to require the most product [24] (Tables 7.3 and 7.4). As the duration of the ECMO course increases, PRBC and platelet transfusion needs are increased as well (Fig. 7.1).

PRBCs

Although a necessary part of ECMO, transfusion of red blood cells is not without risk and potential adverse outcomes. Morbidities associated with red cell transfusion include acute lung injury, transmission of blood-borne infections, central line-associated bloodstream infection, prolonged mechanical ventilation, prolonged hospitalization, and volume overload [16, 30, 34, 52, 60, 61]. Length of an ECMO

Table 7.3 Number of transfusion events during ECMO

		Indication for ECMO			
	Overall	Cardiac	Respiratory	CDH[a]	P-value[b]
RBC, median (mean ± SD)	9 (11.7 ± 7.8)	16 (18.3 ± 13.3)	7 (7.3 ± 3.2)	10 (12.7 ± 6.7)	<0.05
FFP, median (mean ± SD)	5 (5.5 ± 3.7)	5 (6.6 ± 3.5)	4 (3.8 ± 1.8)	5 (6.2 ± 4.2)	<0.05
Platelets, median (mean ± SD)	19 (20.3 ± 11.3)	19 (21.8 ± 10.4)	11 (14.4 ± 8.5)	21 (23.3 ± 12.6)	<0.05
CP, median, (mean) [min-max]	3 (3.7 ± 3.4)	4 (3 ± 1.4)	1 (2.3 ± 2.7)	3 (4.3 ± 3.9)	<0.05

Henríquez-Henríquez [24]
RBC red blood cells, *FFP* fresh frozen plasma, *CP* cryoprecipitate
[a]*P*-values for cardiac indication vs. CDH are not provided since these groups did not differ in any of their requirements
[b]*P*-values correspond to the results of post hoc analysis applied for the following comparisons: respiratory indication vs. cardiac indication and respiratory indication vs. CDH

Table 7.4 Volume requirements of blood components during ECMO

		Indication for ECMO			
	Overall	Cardiac	Respiratory	CDH[a]	P-value[b]
RBC (ml/kg/day). Mean ± SD	35.9 ± 24.7	44.3 ± 31.9	33.1 ± 32.6	35.8 ± 16.6	0.09
FFP (ml/kg/day). Mean	12.9 ± 9.3	16.6 ± 12.1	9.9 ± 7.5	13.7 ± 9.2	<0.05
Platelets (ml/kg/day). Mean	34.3 ± 14.6	33.5 ± 9.5	27.4 ± 12.2	38.4 ± 15.3	<0.05
CP (ml/kg/day). Mean	1.4 ± 2	1.4 ± 1.1	0.5 ± 1	1.9 ± 2.6	<0.05

Henríquez-Henríquez [24]
RBC red blood cells, *FFP* fresh frozen plasma, *CP* cryoprecipitate
[a]*P*-values correspond to the results of post hoc analysis applied for the following comparisons: respiratory indication vs. cardiac indication and respiratory indication vs. CDH
[b]*P*-values for cardiac indication vs. CDH are not provided since these groups did not differ in any of their requirements

course and mortality may be directly associated with the volume of red cell transfusions [26, 53].

Cardiac surgical patients receive the most PRBC transfusions (529 vs. 74 mL/kg for nonsurgical cardiac patients) with median transfusions 131 ml/k/day in cardiac patients and 80 ml/k/day in noncardiac patients in average ECMO runs [21]. Transfusions are given for several reasons during ECMO. One of the initial indications for red cell transfusion is to improve oxygen carrying capacity by maintaining a hematocrit >40. Evaluating the impact of blood transfusion on markers of oxygenation, roughly 5 % of transfusions administered resulted in an increase in SVO2, and 9 % of patients demonstrated an increase in cerebral near-infrared spectroscopy [21]. Other indications for red cell transfusions are anemia secondary to blood loss or hemolysis. PRBC requirements increase the longer a circuit is in use [24]. In patients on ECMO for an average of 9 days, the mean

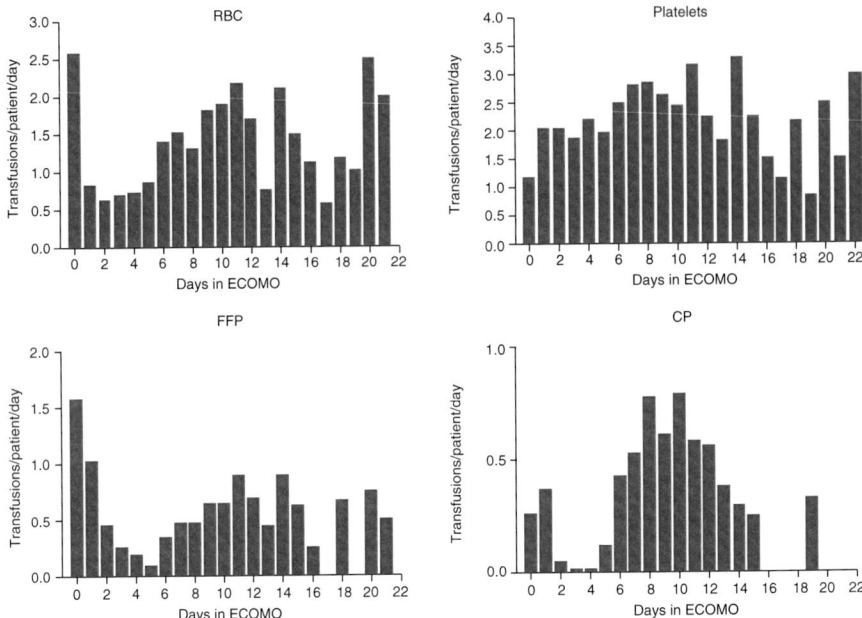

Fig. 7.1 Temporal evolution of transfusion requirements during ECMO. Average number of daily transfusions of red blood (*RBC*), platelets, fresh frozen plasma (*FFP*), and cryoprecipitates (*CP*) per patient (Henríquez-Henríquez [24])

daily transfusion requirements were 39.5 ml/K of PRBC [24]. An aging circuit (>7 days) also increases transfusion needs for red cells as well as plasma and cryoprecipitate. In a dose-dependent manner, red blood cell transfusions are associated with an increase in ECMO days and mortality. Such that with each 10 ml/kg transfusion of red cells, the number of days on ECMO and overall mortality was increased [26, 54].

Fresh (<10-day-old) PRBC is preferred to decrease the chances of potassium leakage and accumulation relative to older units. Washed red cells are utilized across many institutions to minimize the risk of hyperkalemia. However, the use of washed red cells increases the labor associated with preparing a unit of blood and limits its availability for use over time as they expire within 24 h of preparation [62]. Washed cells are also associated with an increased red cell osmotic fragility and risk of hemolysis [37]. For these reasons, the use of washed PRBCs is discouraged if fresh (<10-day-old) PRBCs are available.

The use of CMV-negative and irradiated blood products is a relatively standard practice in neonates. Seronegative, leukocyte-reduced blood decreases CMV transmission risk in immunoincompetent patients (i.e., neonates) who are more likely to demonstrate the clinical manifestation of CMV infection after transfusion. Graft-vs.-host disease occurs when T lymphocytes are transplanted in a host incapable of mounting a response against foreign cells. Gamma irradiation of cellular blood products prevents proliferation of T lymphocytes minimizing the risk of graft-vs.-host disease in the neonates who have an immature immune response.

Blood products containing white cells contribute to negative immunomodulatory effects, infection, and reperfusion injury [1, 44]. Use of non-leuko-reduced red blood cell transfusion has been associated with an increase in mortality in neonatal patients on ECMO [26]. In cardiac surgery and CPB, leukocyte depletion confers benefits in reducing inflammation and reperfusion injury [12].

While many institutions utilize washed, CMV-negative, irradiated, and leuko-reduced blood for neonatal transfusions, some have argued and shown that these precautions may be unwarranted even in the neonatal ECMO population. The gestational ages of the typical neonatal ECMO patient approach term with birth weights >1250 g and are therefore out of the AABB guidelines [1, 38]. However, experience and institutional practice influence the ECMO transfusion practice with the absence of definitive data.

Platelets

The need for platelet transfusion among neonates on ECMO is primarily circuit related due to consumption and dysfunction as well as dependent on the underlying medical diagnosis. No association has been made with length of ECMO and platelet transfusion as seen in PRBCs and FFP [24]. Mean daily platelet transfusion requirement can be 34.3 ml/kg of platelets [24]. The transfusion trigger for platelets varies among institutions and in the literature from 50,000 to 110,000. Some ECMO protocols change platelet parameters over the course of the run (e.g., from 100,000 for the first 3 days to 80,000 after day 3 of ECMO). The average number of platelet transfusions is 1.3–2.2 transfusions per day and is higher on VA compared to VV ECMO [14, 24]. Platelet needs do not appear to be increased with an aging circuit as requirements remain fairly consistent throughout the course with a mean of 2.2 transfusion/day [24]. Platelet transfusions account for the majority of the donor exposures among neonates on ECMO. Average donor exposure per course of ECMO can be significant at 22.8 donors [39]. Significant reductions in donor exposure have been seen in ECMO patients receiving aliquoted apheresis platelets [51].

Plasma

FFP contains the components necessary for coagulation, fibrinolysis, and the complement system as well as proteins required to maintain oncotic pressure and regulate immunity. Plasma is required for preparation of the oxygenator with red cells in the priming process and indicated for the treatment of the complex coagulopathy. In the setting of massive transfusion (>1 blood volume in 24 h) like ECMO, replacement of coagulation factors as well as antithrombin III via FFP becomes necessary. The average use of FFP in neonatal ECMO has been described as high as 12.9 ml/kg/day [24]. Patients with cardiac disease or CDH have higher FFP requirements. FFP use is also increased in an aging circuit [24]. Adverse effects from the administration of plasma include allergic transfusion reactions (ART), transfusion-associated circulatory overload (TACO), and transfusion-related acute lung injury (TRALI), and infections are not common in neonates yet must be considered [47].

Cryoprecipitate

Cryoprecipitate is a frozen blood product prepared from plasma primarily used to replace fibrinogen. Indications in this population are for excessive bleeding from anticoagulation, massive hemorrhage, hypofibrinogenemia (fibrinogen <100–150) related to massive transfusion, and disseminated intravascular coagulation (DIC) [3, 15]. Average daily use in the neonatal ECMO population has been described as 1.4 ml/k/day with a noted increase in CDH/cardiac cases and as the circuit ages [24].

Future State

Institution of protocols for transfusion and anticoagulation management as well as safe modification to transfusion practices and blood component management have been utilized to reduce overall transfusion of products [11, 39, 51]. Routine use of ATIII has been associated with less transfusion of products (PRBCs, platelet, FFP) but needs to be evaluated in a prospective randomized trial [48]. Redefining transfusion parameters, particularly for routine PRBC transfusion, may reduce donor exposure over time as the theoretical benefit of transfusing to a predefine hematocrit to improve oxygenation did not result in an improvement of global measures of oxygenation. This however would benefit from a randomized trial demonstrating equal benefit without an increase in adverse outcomes [21]. Perhaps changes in the circuit components and design may contribute to a reduction of transfusions in neonatal ECMO as they have in CPB and adult ECMO [18, 29, 32].

Anticoagulation Management

Coagulation management is the most challenging part of the care of a neonate on ECMO. A constant balance between clot formation and bleeding needs to be addressed continuously during the ECMO run. Occurring in up to 54 % of ECMO cases, hemorrhagic complications can be devastating and even life threatening [63].

Neonates are susceptible to coagulopathies due to their immature coagulation function, decreased factor levels, and blunted platelet activation, secretion, and aggregation compared to adults [5, 20]. These differences coupled with systemic anticoagulation and ECMO-related platelet consumption and dysfunction, enhanced fibrinolysis, and consumptive coagulopathy result in significantly increased risk for bleeding [63].

Prevention of circuit clots and hemorrhagic complications requires frequent monitoring of coagulation [8, 9, 28]. No single test effectively monitors all factors necessary to determine adequate anticoagulation with heparin [22]. Institutional specific algorithms in conjunction with the ELSO guideline for management of anticoagulation recommend a variety of test to monitor anticoagulation [8, 9, 19].

Activated Clotting Time (ACT)

The most commonly utilized test to monitor unfractionated heparin therapy is the activated clotting time (ACT). It is a whole-blood point-of-care test providing a global assessment of hemostasis. Factors such as anemia, hypofibrinogenemia, thrombocytopenia, platelet dysfunction, coagulation factor deficiencies, elevated D-dimers, hypothermia, and hemodilution can prolong results. Hypercoagulable states can decrease ACT levels [8, 9]. ACT is not a consistent marker of heparin activity and therefore must be used in conjunction with anti-Xa and aPTT to accurately reflect heparin activity [8, 9, 35, 41]. Goal ranges should be maintained 180–240 s. During acute bleeding lowering parameters may be considered for a limited time.

Anti-factor Xa Activity Levels (Anti-Xa)

Anti-Xa is a measure of effect of unfractionated heparin to catalyze antithrombin's inhibition of factor Xa. It does not measure unfractionated heparin concentration and therefore more accurately reflects heparin activity [19]. Specific to unfractionated heparin and not affected by coagulopathy, thrombocytopenia, or hemodilution, like ACT and aPTT, it has been shown to correlate better with heparin dosing [35, 41]. Goal ranges are 0.3–0.7 per ELSO anticoagulation guidelines [19].

Activated Partial Thromboplastin Time (aPTT)

aPTT is a plasma-based test that measures the time to fibrin formation. It is prolonged in infants, but has better correlation with heparin activity compared to ACT [55, 63]. Goal ranges are institution specific [19].

Antithrombin III

Since acquired antithrombin III deficiency is common in neonatal patients requiring ECMO, measurement and replacement during ECMO are beneficial to reduce hemorrhagic complications [42, 48, 57].

Thromboelastography (TEG) and Thromboelastometry (ROTEM)

Thromboelastography is a whole-blood point-of-care test that measures the integrity of the coagulation cascade from fibrin formation to lysis including platelet activity. By testing paired samples, coagulation in the presence of unfractionated heparin can be assessed. It can be useful in evaluating antithrombin need as well as fibrinogen function [19]. Thrombelastograph profiles give an indication of hemostatic states ranging from coagulopathy to hypercoagulability (Table 7.5).

As there is no single gold standard test, a multimodal approach to monitoring appropriate anticoagulation should include a combination of the above testing with a systematic approach or algorithm for interpretation.

Hemorrhagic complications

Hemorrhagic complications are the most frequent complication on ECMO. Hemorrhage on ECMO often is a direct result of the heparinization required to maintain the ECMO circuit. Most commonly, hemorrhage occurs at the surgical site (i.e., cannula site) or at a site of a previous invasive procedure occurring in up to 32 % of patients. Intracranial hemorrhage (ICH) is the most devastating of the hemorrhagic complications on ECMO occurring 7.4–9.9 % of neonates receiving ECMO [23, 25]. In neonates placed on ECMO in the first week of life, the incidence of ICH is inversely proportional to gestational age [54]. It is most likely to occur in patients <30 days old and those requiring cardiac surgery [25]. Other factors include gestational age, acidosis, sepsis, coagulopathy, and receiving epinephrine [23]. Hemorrhagic infarction of CNS and intrathoracic, abdominal, and retroperitoneal bleeding may also occur [7].

Clots in the circuit are the most common mechanical complication. Significant clots can cause oxygenator failure, a consumptive coagulopathy, or pulmonary or systemic emboli. In some centers, heparin-bonded, surface-treated circuits have been used to decrease the frequency of these complications [22].

Table 7.5 Monitoring heparin therapy

Test	Key features	Pros	Cons
Activated clotting time (ACT)	Most commonly utilized test to monitor unfractionated heparin therapy Activator added to whole blood provides global functional assessment of hemostasis Goal ranges maintained 180–240 s	Easily available Whole-blood POC Established norms Familiar Inexpensive	Not a consistent marker of heparin activity Poor correlation with anti-Xa and aPTT Prolonged with anemia, hypofibrinogenemia, thrombocytopenia, platelet dysfunction, coagulation factor deficiencies, elevated D-dimers, hypothermia, and hemodilution Decreased in hypercoagulable states
Activated prothrombin time (aPTT)	Plasma-based test Measures time to fibrin formation Measures activity of intrinsic and common coagulation pathways	Correlates better with heparin activity than ACT Improves with age Long-standing use	Prolonged in neonates No set standard reference ranges Prolonged with factor deficiencies or with lupus anticoagulant Decreased with elevated fibrinogen or factor VIII, particularly in the setting of acute phase reactions Affected by hemodilution Goal ranges are institution specific
Anti-factor Xa activity level	Chromogenic or clot-based assay Measures heparin's ability to catalyze antithrombin inhibition of factor Xa	Current standard for monitoring and adjust heparin and LMWH Not affected by lupus anticoagulant, factor deficiencies, fibrinogen, or FVIII Correlates well with heparin activity	Elevated hemoglobin, bilirubin, or lipids affects assay More expensive than ACT or aPTT Limited studies with current recommendations for therapeutic range (goal ranges are 0.3–0.7)
Thromboelastography and thromboelastometry	Viscoelastic whole-blood analysis of clot formation Measures the integrity of the coagulation cascade from fibrin formation to lysis including platelet activity Using paired tests, heparin activity can be assessed	POC provided continuous assessment of coagulation cascade Use to determine heparin resistance	Complex testing, equipment, and training required for interpretation of results Measures only in vitro clotting not local factors affecting clotting

Adapted from Mok and Lee [40]

Hematologic Considerations

Once bleeding occurs, center-specific transfusion guidelines and clinical status determine transfusion requirements. Transfusion of PRBCs is given to replace blood loss and optimize oxygen delivery, maintaining hematocrit >35%. Due to the ongoing platelet consumption that occurs while on ECMO and given the relationship between platelet count and hemorrhagic complications on ECMO, it is critical to maintain platelets >100,000, particularly in neonates to decrease the degree of bleeding complications. FFP would be warranted in cases of significant bleeding to maintain INR >1.5–2. In cases where ATIII levels are low, use of pooled recombinant ATIII to replenish ATIII levels is beneficial. If fibrinogen levels <100–150 mg/dL, cryoprecipitate may benefit hemostasis. Adjusting the parameters to reduce anticoagulation during acute bleeding is often warranted. If heparin-bonded or surface-treated circuits are used, heparin therapy may temporary be discontinued [4].

Inhibitors of fibrinolysis, such as aminocaproic acid (Amicar), tranexamic acid (TEA), and aprotinin, may be helpful during acute stages of bleeding particularly in the case of surgical bleeding [17]. Case reports describe the use of activated recombinant factor VII for intractable bleeding during ECMO which may have some benefit; however, it must be used cautiously in the setting of ECMO secondary to increase in circuit component clotting as well as the risk of fatal thrombosis [13, 56, 59].

Course and Outcomes

Clear survival benefit for ECMO in neonates with respiratory failure has been demonstrated over the past three decades. The number needed to treat (NNT) for ECMO as a therapy is 4–5, meaning that one additional child survives without severe disability for every four to five children treated with ECMO. Survival rates are the highest for meconium aspiration syndrome (94%) and RDS (84%) [10]. The lowest survival in neonatal ECMO is in the CDH population (51%) and cardiac (40%) with a downward trend over the last decade likely related to increase illness severity. Overall survival is 68% for all comers [4, 46].

Patient-specific hemorrhagic complications that were noted in the ELSO registry were intracranial hemorrhage (7%), bleeding from cannulation site (7.1%), bleeding from surgical sites (6.3%), bleeding from GI tract 1.7%), and pulmonary hemorrhage (4.5%). The presence of one of these complications was associated with significantly lower survival rates between 44 and 64%. The lowest survival overall was seen in cases of intracranial hemorrhage or surgical site bleeding [4].

In terms of long-term outcome, up to 20% of neonates receiving ECMO therapy have neurological complications [40]. Survivors of neonatal ECMO may suffer from subtle neurodevelopmental problems (including behavior) presenting later and becoming more apparent over time [40].

References

1. AABB, Clinical Transfusion Medicine Committee. AABB Committee Report: reducing transfusion-transmitted cytomegalovirus infections. Transfusion. 2016;56(6 Pt 2):1581–7.
2. Anderson HL 3rd, Snedecor S. Multicenter comparison of conventional venoarterial access versus venovenous double-lumen catheter access in newborn infants undergoing extracorporeal membrane oxygenation. J Pediatr Surg. 1993;28(4):530–4.
3. Ang AL, Teo D. Blood transfusion requirements and independent predictors of increased transfusion requirements among adult patients on extracorporeal membrane oxygenation: a single centre experience. Vox Sang. 2009;96(1):34–43.
4. Annich G, Lynch WR, MacLaren G, Wilson JM, Barlett RH, editors. ECMO extracorporeal cardiopulmonary support in critical care. 4th ed. Ann Arbor: ELSO; 2012.
5. Baker-Groberg SM, Lattimore S, et al. Assessment of neonatal platelet adhesion, activation, and aggregation. J Thromb Haemost. 2016;14(4):815–27.
6. Barrett CS, Jaggers JJ, et al. Outcomes of neonates undergoing extracorporeal membrane oxygenation support using centrifugal versus roller blood pumps. Ann Thorac Surg. 2012;94(5):1635–41.
7. Bartlett RH, Roloff DW, et al. Extracorporeal life support: the University of Michigan experience. JAMA. 2000;283(7):904–8.
8. Bembea MM, Annich G, et al. Variability in anticoagulation management of patients on extracorporeal membrane oxygenation: an international survey. Pediatr Crit Care Med. 2013;14(2):e77–84.
9. Bembea MM, Schwartz JM, et al. Anticoagulation monitoring during pediatric extracorporeal membrane oxygenation. ASAIO J. 2013;59(1):63–8.
10. Bennett CC, Johnson A, UK Collaborative ECMO Trial Group. UK collaborative randomised trial of neonatal extracorporeal membrane oxygenation: follow-up to age 4 years. Lancet. 2001;357(9262):1094–6.
11. Bjerke HS, Kelly Jr RE, et al. Decreasing transfusion exposure risk during extracorporeal membrane oxygenation (ECMO). Transfus Med. 1992;2(1):43–9.
12. Boodram S, Evans E. Use of leukocyte-depleting filters during cardiac surgery with cardiopulmonary bypass: a review. J Extra Corpor Technol. 2008;40(1):27–42.
13. Bui JD, Despotis GD, et al. Fatal thrombosis after administration of activated prothrombin complex concentrates in a patient supported by extracorporeal membrane oxygenation who had received activated recombinant factor VII. J Thorac Cardiovasc Surg. 2002;124(4):852–4.
14. Chevuru SC, Sola MC, Florida Collaborative Neonatology Research Group. Multicenter analysis of platelet transfusion usage among neonates on extracorporeal membrane oxygenation. Pediatrics. 2002;109(6):e89.
15. Diab YA, Wong EC, Luban NL. Massive transfusion in children and neonates. Br J Haematol. 2013;161(1):15–26.
16. Dodd RY. Emerging infections, transfusion safety, and epidemiology. N Engl J Med. 2003;349(13):1205–6.
17. Downard CD, Betit P, et al. Impact of AMICAR on hemorrhagic complications of ECMO: a ten-year review. J Pediatr Surg. 2003;38(8):1212–6.
18. Durandy Y. The impact of vacuum-assisted venous drainage and miniaturized bypass circuits on blood transfusion in pediatric cardiac surgery. ASAIO J. 2009;55(1):117–20.
19. ELSO. ELSO Anticoagulation Guidelines. 2016. Retrieved from elso.org: https://www.elso.org/portals/0/files/elsoanticoagulationguideline8-2014-table-contents.pdf.
20. Ferrer-Marin F, Stanworth S, et al. Distinct differences in platelet production and function between neonates and adults: implications for platelet transfusion practice. Transfusion. 2013;53(11):2814–21.

21. Fiser RT, Irby K, et al. RBC transfusion in pediatric patients supported with extracorporeal membrane oxygenation: is there an impact on tissue oxygenation? Pediatr Crit Care Med. 2014;15(9):806–13.
22. Annich GM. Extracorporeal life support: the precarious balance of hemostasis. J Thromb Haemost. 2015;13 Suppl 1:S336–42.
23. Hardart GE, Fackler JC. Predictors of intracranial hemorrhage during neonatal extracorporeal membrane oxygenation. J Pediatr. 1999;134(2):156–9.
24. Henríquez-Henríquez M, Kattan J, et al. Blood component usage during extracorporeal membrane oxygenation: experience in 98 patients at a Latin-American tertiary hospital. Int J Artif Organs. 2014;37(3):233–40.
25. Hervey-Jumper SL, Annich GM. Neurological complications of extracorporeal membrane oxygenation in children. J Neurosurg Pediatr. 2011;7(4):338–44.
26. Jackson HT, Oyetunji TA, et al. The impact of leukoreduced red blood cell transfusion on mortality of neonates undergoing extracorporeal membrane oxygenation. J Surg Res. 2014;192(1):6–11.
27. Karimova A, Brown K, et al. Neonatal extracorporeal membrane oxygenation: practice patterns and predictors of outcome in the UK. Arch Dis Child Fetal Neonatal Ed. 2009;94(2):F129–32.
28. Khaja WA, Bilen O, et al. Evaluation of heparin assay for coagulation management in newborns undergoing ECMO. Am J Clin Pathol. 2010;134(6):950–4.
29. Khoshbin E, Westrope C, et al. Performance of polymethyl pentene oxygenators for neonatal extracorporeal membrane oxygenation: a comparison with silicone membrane oxygenators. Perfusion. 2005;20(3):129–34.
30. Kipps AK, Wypij D, et al. Blood transfusion is associated with prolonged duration of mechanical ventilation in infants undergoing reparative cardiac surgery. Pediatr Crit Care Med. 2011;12(1):52–6.
31. Krisa VM, Kevin L, Peek G, Joseph Z, editors. ECMO extracorporeal cardiopulmonary support in critical care. 3rd ed. Ann Arbor: ELSO; 2005.
32. Kulat B, Zingle N. Optimizing circuit design using a remote-mounted perfusion system. J Extra Corpor Technol. 2009;41(1):28–31.
33. Lequier L, Horton SB, et al. Extracorporeal membrane oxygenation circuitry. Pediatr Crit Care Med. 2013;14(5 Suppl 1):S7–12.
34. Li G, Rachmale S, et al. Incidence and transfusion risk factors for transfusion-associated circulatory overload among medical intensive care unit patients. Transfusion. 2011;51(2): 338–43.
35. Liveris A, Bello RA, et al. Anti-factor Xa assay is a superior correlate of heparin dose than activated partial thromboplastin time or activated clotting time in pediatric extracorporeal membrane oxygenation. Pediatr Crit Care Med. 2014;15(2):e72–9.
36. Madar J, Richmond S. Role of extracorporeal membrane oxygenation. Lancet. 1996;348(9030):823–4.
37. Masalunga C, Cruz M, et al. Increased hemolysis from saline pre-washing RBCs or centrifugal pumps in neonatal ECMO. J Perinatol. 2007;27(6):380–4.
38. McCoy-Pardington D, Judd WJ, et al. Blood use during extracorporeal membrane oxygenation. Transfusion. 1990;30(4):307–9.
39. Minifee PK, et al. Decreasing blood donor exposure in neonates on extracorporeal membrane oxygenation. J Pediatr Surg. 1990;25(1):38–42.
40. Mok YH, Lee J. Neonatal extracorporeal membrane oxygenation: update on management strategies and long-term outcomes. Adv Neonatal Care. 2016;16(1):26–36.
41. Nankervis CA, Preston TJ, et al. Assessing heparin dosing in neonates on venoarterial extracorporeal membrane oxygenation. ASAIO J. 2007;53(1):111–4.
42. Niebler RA, Christensen M, et al. Antithrombin replacement during extracorporeal membrane oxygenation. Artif Organs. 2011;35(11):1024–8.
43. Luban NL. Neonatal red blood cell transfusions. Vox Sang. 2004;87 Suppl 2:184–8.

44. Ortolano GA, Aldea GS, et al. A review of leukofiltration in cardiac surgery: the time course of reperfusion injury may facilitate study design of anti-inflammatory effects. Perfusion. 2002;17(Suppl):53–62.
45. Osiovich HC, Peliowski A, et al. The Edmonton experience with venovenous extracorporeal membrane oxygenation. J Pediatr Surg. 1998;33(12):1749–52.
46. Paden ML, Paden ML, Rycus PL, Thiagarajan PR, ELSO Registry. Update and outcomes in extracorporeal life support. Semin Perinatol. 2014;38(2):65–70.
47. Pandey S, Vyas GN. Adverse effects of plasma transfusion. Transfusion. 2012;52 Suppl 1:65S–79.
48. Perry R, Stein J, et al. Antithrombin III administration in neonates with congenital diaphragmatic hernia during the first three days of extracorporeal membrane oxygenation. J Pediatr Surg. 2013;48(9):1837–42.
49. Polito A, Barrett CS, et al. Neurologic complications in neonates supported with extracorporeal membrane oxygenation. An analysis of ELSO registry data. Intensive Care Med. 2013;39(9):1594–601.
50. Qureshi FG, Jackson HT, et al. The changing population of the United States and use of extracorporeal membrane oxygenation. J Surg Res. 2013;184(1):572–6.
51. Rosenberg EM, Chambers LA, et al. A program to limit donor exposures to neonates undergoing extracorporeal membrane oxygenation. Pediatrics. 1994;94(3):341–6.
52. Salvin JW, Scheurer MA, et al. Blood transfusion after pediatric cardiac surgery is associated with prolonged hospital stay. Ann Thorac Surg. 2011;91(1):204–10.
53. Smith A, Hardison D, et al. Red blood cell transfusion volume and mortality among patients receiving extracorporeal membrane oxygenation. Perfusion. 2013;28(1):54–60.
54. Smith KM, McMullan DM, et al. Is age at initiation of extracorporeal life support associated with mortality and intraventricular hemorrhage in neonates with respiratory failure? J Perinatol. 2014;34(5):386–91.
55. Sulkowski JP, Preston TJ, et al. Comparison of routine laboratory measures of heparin anticoagulation for neonates on extracorporeal membrane oxygenation. J Extra Corpor Technol. 2014;46(1):69–76.
56. Syburra T, Lachat M, et al. Fatal outcome of recombinant factor VIIa in heart transplantation with extracorporeal membrane oxygenation. Ann Thorac Surg. 2010;89(5):1643–5.
57. Urlesberger B, Zobel G, et al. Activation of the clotting system during extracorporeal membrane oxygenation in term newborn infants. J Pediatr. 1996;129(2):264–8.
58. Usher R, Shephard M, Lind J. The blood volume of the newborn infant and placental transfusion. Acta Paediatr. 1963;52:497–512.
59. Velik-Salchner C, Sergi C. Use of recombinant factor VIIa (Novoseven) in combination with other coagulation products led to a thrombotic occlusion of the truncus brachiocephalicus in a neonate supported by extracorporeal membrane oxygenation. Anesth Analg. 2005;101(3):924.
60. Vlaar AP, Binnekade JM, et al. Risk factors and outcome of transfusion-related acute lung injury in the critically ill: a nested case–control study. Crit Care Med. 2010;38(3):771–8.
61. Wylie MC, Graham DA, et al. Risk factors for central line-associated bloodstream infection in pediatric intensive care units. Infect Control Hosp Epidemiol. 2010;31(10):1049–56.
62. Yuan S, Tsukahara E, et al. How we provide transfusion support for neonatal and pediatric patients on extracorporeal membrane oxygenation. Transfusion. 2013;53(6):1157–65.
63. Zavadil DP, Stammers AH, et al. Hematological abnormalities in neonatal patients treated with extracorporeal membrane oxygenation (ECMO). J Extra Corpor Technol. 1998;30(2):83–90.

Index

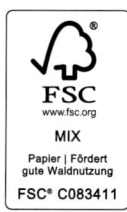

Zeitfracht Medien GmbH
Ferdinand-Jühlke-Straße 7
99095 Erfurt, Deutschland
produktsicherheit@kolibri360.de